How to Promote Wellbeing

How to Promote Wellbeing

Practical Steps for Healthcare Practitioners' Mental Health

Dr Rachel K. Thomas
Central and North West London
NHS Foundation Trust
UK

WILEY Blackwell

Registered Office(s)
John Wiley & Sons, Inc., 111 River Street, Hoboken, NJ 07030, USA
John Wiley & Sons Ltd, The Atrium, Southern Gate, Chichester, West Sussex, PO19 8SQ, UK

Editorial Office
9600 Garsington Road, Oxford, OX4 2DQ, UK

For details of our global editorial offices, customer services, and more information about Wiley products visit us at www.wiley.com.

Wiley also publishes its books in a variety of electronic formats and by print-on-demand. Some content that appears in standard print versions of this book may not be available in other formats.

Limit of Liability/Disclaimer of Warranty
The contents of this work are intended to further general scientific research, understanding, and discussion only and are not intended and should not be relied upon as recommending or promoting scientific method, diagnosis, or treatment by physicians for any particular patient. In view of ongoing research, equipment modifications, changes in governmental regulations, and the constant flow of information relating to the use of medicines, equipment, and devices, the reader is urged to review and evaluate the information provided in the package insert or instructions for each medicine, equipment, or device for, among other things, any changes in the instructions or indication of usage and for added warnings and precautions. While the publisher and authors have used their best efforts in preparing this work, they make no representations or warranties with respect to the accuracy or completeness of the contents of this work and specifically disclaim all warranties, including without limitation any implied warranties of merchantability or fitness for a particular purpose. No warranty may be created or extended by sales representatives, written sales materials or promotional statements for this work. The fact that an organization, website, or product is referred to in this work as a citation and/or potential source of further information does not mean that the publisher and authors endorse the information or services the organization, website, or product may provide or recommendations it may make. This work is sold with the understanding that the publisher is not engaged in rendering professional services. The advice and strategies contained herein may not be suitable for your situation. You should consult with a specialist where appropriate. Further, readers should be aware that websites listed in this work may have changed or disappeared between when this work was written and when it is read. Neither the publisher nor authors shall be liable for any loss of profit or any other commercial damages, including but not limited to special, incidental, consequential, or other damages.

Library of Congress Cataloging-in-Publication Data

Names: Thomas, Rachel K. (Rachel Katherine), author.
Title: How to promote wellbeing : practical steps for healthcare
    practitioners' mental health / Rachel K. Thomas.
Description: First edition. | Hoboken, NJ : Wiley-Blackwell, 2021. |
    Includes index.
Identifiers: LCCN 2020032172 (print) | LCCN 2020032173 (ebook) | ISBN
    9781119614364 (paperback) | ISBN 9781119614395 (adobe pdf) | ISBN
    9781119614401 (epub)
Subjects: MESH: Health Promotion–methods | Mental Health | Mental
    Disorders–prevention & control | Stress, Psychological–prevention &
    control | Global Health
Classification: LCC RC455 (print) | LCC RC455 (ebook) | NLM WM 101 | DDC
    616.89–dc23
LC record available at https://lccn.loc.gov/2020032172
LC ebook record available at https://lccn.loc.gov/20200321

Cover Design: Wiley
Cover Image: © TECHDESIGNWORK/Getty Images

Set in 9.5/12pt Minion by SPi Global, Pondicherry, India
Printed and bound by CPI Group (UK) Ltd, Croydon, CR0 4YY

10 9 8 7 6 5 4 3 2 1

Contents

About the author

Dr Rachel Thomas is a medical doctor in the NHS, in central London. She is the award-winning author of books including *Practical Medical Procedures at a Glance*, and *Medical School at a Glance*, and is the founder of the mental health platform *the wellbeing doctor*. She has a medical degree from the University of Oxford, and an MSc in the neuroscience and psychology of mental health from King's College London. She also holds a BSc and a BEng in Biomedical Engineering from the University of Sydney.

Acknowledgements

Thank you to those who have supported this book.

Great thanks go to Dr Diana Thomas for her invaluable assistance with all aspects of this book. Thanks also go to Hugh, Rob, Matthew, Pepper, Camilla, Peter, Sienna, Andrew, James, Alyssa, and Napoleon for their support.

Thanks go to the various healthcare practitioners that have kindly had input into this book. In particular, thanks go to Lara Lopes de Jesus, counselling psychologist, for her feedback.

Thanks also go to James Watson, Anne Hunt, and Tom Marriott at Wiley Blackwell Publishing for turning this book into a reality, at a time when the mental health and wellbeing of clinicians – indeed that of us all - is being so significantly tested.

Preface

This book provides a concise resource for addressing many mental health and wellbeing challenges that we, as clinicians, may be confronted with. These are summarised in an evidence-based toolkit to help us in several ways. Initially, to decrease the risk and impact of potentially debilitating conditions such as burnout on ourselves, and consequently, to impact more positively on our patients' outcomes.

Working in healthcare means that we are at the helm of an unsteady ship, a system focussed on providing optimal care for patients. We have to be ready to act when required – be this at 2am on a night shift, on a long weekend day shift with skeleton staff, or in the middle of a day when we can feel our blood sugar dropping to our boots as the imaginary idea of lunch hour sails by. Unfortunately, keeping an even keel is often at the sacrifice of those of us working within this system.

Emergencies are unpredictable. Patients can suddenly deteriorate. Someone who seems on the mend one moment, can be seriously ill the next, for example with infections or complications. Coupled with immune systems that are already under pressure, the results can swiftly become catastrophic. And when the unthinkable happens and a pandemic sweeps the globe, the cases of emergencies and deteriorations start to occur at an exponential rate. Healthcare systems are expanded to cope in as best a way as they can, stretching all of their components, including clinicians working within them, to breaking point and beyond.

The idea that clinicians suffer from 'injury', such as burnout, due to an overstretched healthcare system is increasingly becoming apparent. The COVID-19 crisis has highlighted how our healthcare systems need to protect not only the patients, but also the clinicians and other healthcare practitioners working within the system.

While positive steps towards improving mental health and wellbeing for the general population are being taken, such as increased conversation and decreased stigma around mental health and wellbeing, this progress has arguably not translated to clinicians. Research reveals that mental health conditions are increasing in this group, and that these conditions may be exacerbated by perceived reluctance or delay in seeking additional help and support. Conditions such as burnout and injury may not be due to failures in the individual clinician, but rather more due to factors such as excessive workloads, workplace culture, or overall work environment.

The importance of the wellbeing of clinicians is being increasingly recognised. However, although well-intentioned advice to support us may be given, this may seem impractical at the times when it is needed most. Some of this advice may seem tone-deaf to the real-world practicalities of when we are 'on the job'. This is not to say that the role of people in different fields in helping to protect and preserve our mental health and wellbeing is unhelpful. Quite the contrary. We need people who have a more objective view of what a work–life balance is, to help many of us in healthcare roles who have long-forgotten the concept, albeit through no fault of our own. This slow erosion of our work–life balance often starts early in our training. The sheer quantity of knowledge we are required to digest and retain, the stress of exams, and the very nature of the areas we are training to become proficient in, can leave us with a different perspective of what work is, what life is, and how, exactly are we to balance the two.

A hospital I once worked in had a brightly coloured poster informing us of ways to decrease our stress. The poster had 10 small sketches, with information added in artistic calligraphy. Each suggestion was sensible, and indeed even likely to be very useful in many occupations. However, healthcare often isn't just any regular profession. At times, suggestions to leave work on time, and to make sure we take our lunch breaks, are practically impossible. If a hand-over is needed, we cannot leave until this is done, no matter whose birthday dinner we are missing – even if it is our own.

It is recognised that, as clinicians, we have conflicting pressures at times. Historically, delivering high quality patient care along with maintaining our own personal health and wellbeing were often perceived as being at odds with each other – that pausing for ourselves meant neglecting patients. However, it is time for us to challenge these historical views in light of evidence showing we need to, as the airline safety videos so succinctly phrase it, 'put on our own oxygen mask first', in order to continue to deliver and perform optimally throughout our career. This has never been more acutely highlighted than during the COVID-19 pandemic, where, due to forces beyond our control, our inability to always put on our own mask first – literally – led to sacrifices not only of wellbeing, but of life.

While highlighting many of the benefits, and our sense of pride, in the healthcare system's responsiveness as a whole, the COVID-19 pandemic has also highlighted areas for improvement, and stimulated discussion on how this could be achieved.

Research increasingly supports evidence of the significant links between mental and physical health. Evidence suggests that patients with mental health issues are more likely to have physical health issues, leading to poorer health outcomes. For instance, it has been shown that patients with cardiovascular disease are also more likely to have depression, when compared to the rest of the general population.[1] Conversely, there is also evidence that people with depression are more likely to develop cardiovascular disease, when compared to those who are not depressed.[1] So it is important to take a patient's mental health into consideration when evaluating their physical health, as this may lead to a better outcome overall. Additionally, in turn, better outcomes for the patient may link to better outcomes for us, their healthcare practitioners.

The information in this book is relevant to clinicians and other healthcare practitioners – doctors, nurses, dentists, physiotherapists, counsellors, therapists, and other associated team members. Reading it may count towards our continuing professional development points. Combining the suggested strategies with elements of reflection will assist us in promoting and strengthening our own mental health and wellbeing – in turn, in helping us to deliver optimal outcomes for our patients.

During the COVID-19 pandemic, we worked in a healthcare system that responded flexibly to the demands placed upon it. We were called to work in different areas and in different ways, while the infrastructure around us also changed. New hospitals were built and staffed within days in the UK and USA, highlighting the flexibility for a rapid response within the system. However, it also highlighted a period of potential need for increased support for healthcare practitioners. Embracing this newly-found flexibility, we can now consider creating a more balanced set-point for how our healthcare system works, with an increased focus on the mental health and wellbeing of the clinicians who work within it.

Introduction

As clinicians, we are trained to focus on improving the health of our patients. However, this focus, due to numerous reasons, can become so singular that we neglect to look after ourselves.

Healthcare is an extremely rewarding profession. Its capacity to be varied, intense, and emotional offers challenge and high personal satisfaction. The opportunity to help a fellow human at their most vulnerable is a great honour.

However, being a clinician also comes with stress and pressure. The pressures of such a job – and really, for many of us, it becomes more than just a 'job' – come from endless sources. Some pressures are due to systemic, institutional, and organisational aspects, baked into the hospital infrastructure, such as rota hours. Some are cultural, such as the stigma still remaining of mentioning our own mental health issues, where we are part of a profession many people assume is immune from such problems. Education and awareness may be sources of pressure, when appropriate resources are not clear, or even available. In times of crisis, the stress may be operational, such as an increased stretching of teams, inadequate support, or inadequate supplies of personal protective equipment (PPE). Hence, while, unfortunately, many areas may cause stress and pressure, these fortunately also provide many opportunities to improve the situation.

It is not surprising, then, that the accumulation of these factors, compounded by our inherent obligation of responsibility for other people's lives on a daily basis, leads to a profession in which there are high rates of burnout and mental distress.

The impact of burnout and mental distress can lead to immeasurable cost, not only to our own health but, ironically, also to the health of those we are aiming to help. In many studies, clinicians' decreased wellbeing is associated with poorer patient outcomes. Poorer patient outcomes are associated with decreased job enjoyment – which ultimately may lead to more clinicians

How to Promote Wellbeing: Practical Steps for Healthcare Practitioners' Mental Health,
First Edition. Dr Rachel K. Thomas.
© 2021 Dr Rachel K. Thomas. Published 2021 by John Wiley & Sons Ltd.

leaving due to burnout. This leads to fewer clinicians, and it is not hard to see that this can then lead to a compounding effect with even greater stretching of resources and fewer clinicians available. So, in being too devoted to our profession, we may instead actually be undercutting our main priority – our commitment to helping our patients.

This book addresses issues in a direct, practical way, since we, as clinicians, are generally time-poor. In the first half of the book we analyse and highlight problem factors that potentially affect our mental health and wellbeing. Given that our own mental health and wellbeing has the potential to impact on the outcomes of our patients, we then consider the problem factors and protective factors relevant to the mental health and wellbeing specifically of our patients. This is in no way intended to be a complete analysis of this huge area. It is just intended to highlight some areas, and to propose some protective factors that may be of benefit to our patients. The second half of the book provides information on protective factors for clinicians, for preserving our own mental health and wellbeing. Evidence-based tools and techniques are included, for use to not only promote and protect our own wellbeing, but in the process, to enable the continued delivery of optimum levels of care to our patients.

Learning outcomes

- Increased understanding of:
  a. global problems affecting mental health and wellbeing
  b. organisational problem factors affecting mental health and wellbeing
  c. individual problem factors affecting mental health and wellbeing
  d. the impacts of chronic stress
  e. the impacts of burnout
  f. protective factors affecting mental health and wellbeing
- Increased ability to recognise the signs of burnout
- Increased awareness of:
  a. protective factors for promoting organisational resilience
  b. protective factors for promoting individual resilience
  c. the need for recovery behaviours, and potentially suitable behaviours.

Reading this book and then appropriately reflecting on aspects such as the above learning outcomes may qualify as being eligible for Continuing Professional Development (CPD) points. It is also important to note that this book is not intended as a support for us when we are in acute phases of distress or suffering with a mental health condition. The resources in Chapter 7 provide sources of help in any acute instance, as this book is not intended as an exclusive treatment or diagnostic tool. In situations where we are unsure whether we need further help, a conversation with a trusted colleague, local General Practitioner (GP), friend, or family member is a helpful first step.

Why should we be concerned about our own wellbeing?

Healthcare is evidence-based. We use evidence to decide the best treatments and courses of actions for our patients. Why should we not apply the same standard to look after our own wellbeing? Looking at the evidence – as we do in other areas of healthcare – there is plenty to support the fact that we are in the best position to look after our patients when we also look after our own wellbeing.

Grim statistics highlight what happens when we don't.

In the UK, it is estimated that, per year, errors cost the NHS over 1 billion GBP in litigation, and 2 billion GBP due to bed delays.[1] The human cost – grief, pain, and suffering by those at both ends of the error – is, of course, inestimable.

Even if we think we do not have time to care for our own wellbeing, or that it is 'optional', clinician codes of conduct make it clear that maintaining our own wellbeing is essentially a requirement.

Professional codes for different healthcare practitioners cover aspects of practice, and these can be interpreted to either explicitly or implicitly direct us to ensure our own health and wellbeing is adequate.

The General Medical Council (GMC) provides guidelines on ethical guidance and good medical practice.[2] Patient care is the first concern under 'Knowledge, Skills, and Performance'. Associated with *'providing a good standard of practice and care'* is the recognition that we work within our own competence and its limitations.[3]

It even explicitly covers *'risks posed by your health'*.[4] Knowing, or even suspecting, that our performance and/or our judgement could be impacted by a condition requires us to consult with a suitably qualified colleague. While at times we may not be fully aware of how our wellbeing is impacting on us, usually we have at least some degree of insight and self-awareness which means we at least do 'have a hunch' that we may be in need of help.

Taking this a step further means that we should, in all likelihood, take as many steps as possible to protect our mental wellbeing.

The GMC's guide for *'Good Medical Practice'* emphasises that our first concern is the patient's care, and that we should act promptly if we feel this may be compromised. We must monitor the quality of our work, and ensure that we work within the limitations of our competence (Figure 0.1).

The Nursing and Midwifery Council (NMC) outlines professional requirements and standards for nurses in the UK.[5] Nurses joining this register are required to commit to uphold the standards it outlines. The register clearly

knowledge, skills & performance
make the care of your patient your first concern
provide a good standard of practice and care
keep your professional knowledge and skills up to date
recognise and work within the limits of your competence

safety & quality
take prompt action if you think that patient safety, dignity or comfort
is being compromised
protect and promote the health of patients and the public

communication, partnership & teamwork
treat patients as individuals and respect their dignity
treat patients politely and considerately
respect patients' right to confidentiality
work in partnership with patients
listen to, and respond to, their concerns and preferences
give patients the information they want or need in a way they can understand
respect patients' right to reach decisions with you about their treatment and care
support patients in caring for themselves to improve and maintain their health
work with colleagues in the ways that best serve patients' interests

maintaining trust
be honest and open and act with integrity
never discriminate unfairly against patients or colleagues
never abuse your patients' trust in you or the public's trust in the profession

Figure 0.1   Duties of a doctor registered with the GMC.[3]

states that 'nurses, midwives, and nursing associates are expected to work within the limits of their competence'.[5]

The register also clearly states there is a requirement to:

- 'pay special attention to promoting wellbeing, preventing ill health, and meeting the changing health and care needs of people during all life stages

- be supportive of colleagues who are encountering health or performance problems. However, this support must never compromise or be at the expense of patient or public safety

- take account of your own personal safety as well as the safety of people in your care

- take all reasonable personal precautions necessary to avoid any potential health risks to colleagues, people receiving care, and the public

- maintain the level of health you need to carry out your professional role

- *support any staff you may be responsible for to follow the Code at all times. They must have the knowledge, skills, and competence for safe practice; and understand how to raise any concerns linked to any circumstances where the Code has, or could be, broken.*[5]

It can clearly be seen that these, and additional, areas of the code highlight that there is a professional requirement to maintain our own wellbeing. It is not only doctors and nurses who are bound by these requirements. Other healthcare professionals may have similar codes, highlighting the need to ensure and maintain personal wellbeing.

The practice standards are clear for all Allied Health professionals, for example Speech and Language Pathologists, Occupational therapists, Physiotherapists, Physical Therapists, Chiropodists, Audiologists, Diagnostic Imaging Technologists, Specialist Diagnostic Imaging Technologists, Medical Laboratory Technicians, Emergency Medicine Technicians, Addiction Counsellors, and Dietitians.[6]

In the section on 'Maintaining fitness to practice', the standards instruct that an Allied Health professional is to '*maintain his/her own health and wellbeing. A registered professional should restrict or accommodate practice if he/she cannot safely perform essential functions of his/her professional role due to mental or physical disabilities*',[6] to '*strive to maintain a healthy work-life balance*',[6] and that '*registered health professionals should support the health and wellbeing of their colleagues. When doing so a registered professional should encourage colleagues who require care to seek appropriate help*'.[6] Thus, there are clear requirements to look after our own wellbeing, and to ensure we have a work–life balance that is healthy and sustainable.

Hence, it is essential for us to protect our own wellbeing, in order to be able to provide the highest quality of care to our patients. This, in itself, is sufficient motivation. Besides, if we are unwell, we, ourselves, may become a burden on the very healthcare system we are trying to uphold – and negatively impact on workloads, both our own and our colleagues. In any event, by signing up to as clinicians and other healthcare professionals, we have already agreed in principle to protect our own wellbeing through our relevant codes of conduct and ethics.

Why should we consider both problem factors and protective factors?

'Mental health' and 'wellbeing' appear, on the surface, to be influenced by somewhat nebulous factors. Without teasing these factors out, it is difficult to know how to start tackling them. We can give ourselves a 'road map' to follow by categorising the factors as either problem or protective. We then have

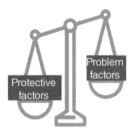

Figure 0.2   Balancing problem and protective factors.

indications of where and how we should direct our attention. There are some problem factors that will always be present, just as there are some protective factors which will never be adequate. With increased awareness, we can start tipping the scales into more balance than has historically been the case, resulting in overall improvement in our mental health and wellbeing (Figure 0.2).

Being physically fit will not categorically prevent illness, and similarly, improving mental resilience and stress management will not categorically avoid burnout. The techniques suggested in this book are useful tools to employ to try to help prevent burnout. These techniques are not a 'cure all', and by using them, all stress and burnout may not necessarily be avoided. If we are unable to avoid burnout, it may not necessarily be due to not having taken enough steps, or not having carried them out assiduously enough. As with physical illness, increasing physical fitness and improving lifestyle aspects, such as nutrition, improve the chances of returning to 'normal functioning' after physical illness and treatment, and decrease the chances of falling ill in the first place. So, too, may the steps in this book improve our chances of strengthening our resilience and if stressed, returning to mental wellness; and potentially decrease our chances of succumbing to stress in the first place.

When the cost of doing nothing is so high, what have we got to lose?

Chapter 1 **General problem factors affecting global mental health and wellbeing**

While our individual mental health and wellbeing are influenced by many factors, so too is that of the overall state of mental health across the globe. The following overview provides a lens through which we can reflect on key aspects.

Problem factor: Global mental health burden

The global burden of mental health conditions is greater than both cancer and cardiovascular disease.[1] Approximately a third of adult health problems and disability across the globe is due to mental illness challenges.[2] Such an enormous global burden has meant that finding solutions to the problem has become a key priority in many countries. The emphasis is now increasingly on potential preventative measures and early, lighter touch interventions, more than ever before.

The average time to treatment after mental health symptoms first appear has been estimated as 10 years, and that two out of every three people who are depressed will not receive care that is adequate.[3] This global crisis has prompted many conversations, as well action plans from institutions such as the World Health Organisation (WHO).

Conversations on mental health issues concerning the general population, a useful starting point for addressing the mental health burden, are increasing in the community. However, these conversations are lagging when it comes to clinicians reflecting on mental health issues in themselves. It is ironic that we instigate and support such conversations, yet – for various reasons as we will discuss – are left with either little insight, or little capacity, for action in regard to *ourselves*.

With these conversations about both the general population and clinicians alike, it is key to remember that mental health conditions are not the fault of the person who is affected by them. Much as we do not blame someone with asthma for having it, we need to ensure that conversations on mental health

How to Promote Wellbeing: Practical Steps for Healthcare Practitioners' Mental Health,
First Edition. Dr Rachel K. Thomas.

issues – be they involving clinicians or not – do not implicitly blame the person who is affected.

Being affected by stress, burnout, or any other mental health condition
is not the fault of the person who is affected.

Burnout, or suffering under the effects of stress, or any other mental health condition, are not due to personal shortcomings and are not due to a failure of some sort in the individual who is affected – whether they are a clinician or not. While this may seem common sense to some of us, on reflection, it may give pause for thought for others.

Burnout can be regarded as a 'fracture' or a reaching of 'breaking point', and it is important to remember that stress can leave 'injury' as it nudges us closer to this point. Just because we have not yet reached breaking point, doesn't mean that we aren't being 'injured' by the stress. And just because we haven't been diagnosed with a mental health condition, doesn't mean that, at times, our mental health is suffering.

Or that our mental health couldn't be improved.

We spend a significant proportion of our lives working. 'Workplace stress' is a common concept in many workplaces, with significant cost associated with many large corporations' efforts to provide wellbeing tools and support for their staff. Acknowledging the impact of stress from work is thus not dissimilar to that which most of our fellow humans are feeling. Recognised sources of stress in a general workplace include:

- A lack of support
- Unrealistic demands
- A lack of appreciation
- An imbalance between effort and reward.[4]

Working as clinicians, we find that these sources of stress are all too common in our areas of work, too. Yet while it is generally acknowledged that working as a clinician is stressful, the support tools that other occupations are provided with are often lacking for us. Particularly within the existing hospital system of many countries, the stresses of work are also related to the infrastructure that we are working within. They may be due to a range of factors, including excessive workloads, a workplace culture that is unsupportive of lowering stress at work, and other aspects of the overall work environment.

In times of crisis, efforts to expand the healthcare system lead to increases in these stresses. Doctors being moved to areas of practice where they have lesser familiarity working in – some even returning from retirement – leads to increases in stress. Inadequate personal protective equipment (PPE) and staffing rotas lead to clinicians being put in positions that can harm not only their own health but that of their patients, too. There is often an 'all systems go' approach to handling crises, while the 'recovery' or 'debrief' phases of such times are often viewed as being less important. After periods at war, the returned servicemen and women have current practice guidelines for debriefing techniques.[5] Given their exposure to death and suffering during their work, it is well recognised that some kind of support will benefit them once they return. We, as clinicians, are also constantly surrounded by death and suffering and may be physically and mentally stretched beyond our coping resources. We are trained to manage both patients and our feelings about their health in times of crisis, but perhaps current practice guidelines should afford us similar support. Reflecting on the support offered in corporate environments may highlight that mental health education and stress management support is offered more extensively there, too, than it is for healthcare professionals.

Our conversations on wellbeing and mental health need to start focussing more on organisational change. However, since organisational change tends to evolve slowly, it may be useful for us to 'put on our own oxygen mask first', as the airline safety videos so aptly phrase it, and learn a few techniques that may help ourselves to relieve the situation on a personal level, until the required systemic changes are eventually implemented. Part of this 'top down' change can begin with a 'bottom up' approach: learning and implementing techniques on a personal level will contribute to the required attitude and institutional changes further up in the system.

It may well be that, given the significant burden of mental health across the globe, our global approach to how it is managed needs to be reviewed. Whether it is increased education in school systems or increased access to telehealth resources – there are multiple avenues for improvement. Maybe the most effective remedies will prove to be institutional as well as personal; only time will tell. In the meantime, however, we clinicians tend to, by necessity, be practical and solution focused. We also tend to appreciate an approach with different and complementary prongs – a multi-disciplinary team approach. While reflecting on greater policy change, it makes sense to reflect not only on some of the wide issues relating to our wellbeing, but also on some of the solutions.

Problem factor: Accessing resources

The issue of the lack of adequate resources for mental health and wellbeing is universal. Across the globe 70% of the general population with a mental illness do not receive any treatment from trained healthcare staff (Figure 1.1).[6] The reasons for this are multiple and complex; however, they include:

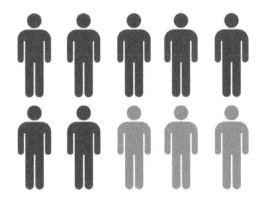

Figure 1.1 Around 7 in 10 of the general population across the globe with a mental illness do not receive any treatment from trained healthcare staff.[6]

- Ignorance of presenting signs and symptoms
- Ignorance of treatment access pathways
- Perception around mental health
- Concerns about being discriminated against.[2]

Approximately one-third of global adult disability is due to issues surrounding mental health.[2] So sobering are these statistics that bodies such as the WHO have responded with 'Mental Health Action Plan' directives.[2] These include:

- More effective leadership and governance for mental health
- The provision of comprehensive, integrated mental health and social care services in community-based settings
- Implementation of strategies for promotion and prevention
- Strengthened information systems, evidence, and research.[7]

As mentioned, evidence suggests that it may take almost a decade for treatment to begin for depression after depressed symptoms have first appeared.[2] There is also evidence that delays in health professionals seeking treatment are greater than those of the general population. Hence the statistics for us and our colleagues could clearly be improved.

There are a range of different care options for mental health. While traditional face-to-face consultations with a trained clinician are key in some cases, there are a range of other, potentially more accessible treatment options that may be suitable in some cases. Some may include telemedicine, or complementary and alternative treatments. While some of these are in relative infancy, their potential is promising. Internet-based cognitive behavioural therapy programmes aim to teach both cognitive skills – such as identifying depressogenic biases in how information is being processed – and behavioural skills, such as strategies to solve problems.

> *A range of factors may delay clinicians
> accessing mental health and wellbeing resources.*

Clinicians also may delay access to care due to concerns around confidentiality.[8] There are other factors affecting how and why we access support in the way we do, as we will cover in the coming chapters.

Problem factor: Multiple potential impacts on individual mental health

The biopsychosocial (BPS) model framework is used to explore how a mental health condition has arisen.[9] The BPS model outlines the broad scope of areas that impact on our mental health, and systematically shows their inter-connections. According to this framework, there are various interconnected components that contribute to mental health conditions. These include the biological, the psychological, and the social. It shows that social parameters, the surrounding personality, and our emotional tone, as well as many other aspects all influence our mental health.[10]

Some factors include (Figure 1.2):

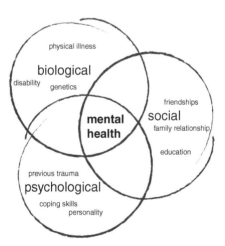

Figure 1.2 The biopsychosocial model indicates the interconnectedness between biological, psychological, and social factors that influence mental health.

- Biological: age, genetics, gender, disability, co-morbid disease
- Psychological: beliefs, attitudes, self-perception, self-esteem, coping skills
- Social: friendships, occupation, employment, family relationships, social support systems, socioeconomics.

Some of these aspects are modifiable; for example coping skills are highly modifiable.

Neurobiology and genomics research provide strong evidence on the complexity of the expression of mental health conditions. A simple, linear cause and effect model rarely, if ever, can explain a mental health condition. Instead, it is more like a looping and complex chain of multiple causes and effects.[10]

In recognising areas that impact on our mental health, we can identify those that we can improve in order to help protect and promote our mental health. Therefore, this framework presents a way to not only look at factors that negatively affect our mental health, but to also highlight areas that contribute positively to our mental health.

Problem factor: The acute and chronic stress responses

As many of us are aware, our stress responses can be acute (quicker and shorter) or chronic (over a longer timeframe). Research supports that the implications of stress can extend beyond our physical health to our mental health, too.

An acute stress response follows the perception of a stressful event, and leads to changes in the

- Endocrine
- Cardiovascular
- Nervous
- Immune

systems.[11] These changes, known as the 'acute stress response', or the 'fight or flight' response, are, when short in duration, important adaptations for our survival.

Chemical cascades are generally activated (Figure 1.3) to:

- Release energy stores for immediately available use
- Distribute energy to tissues – such as the brain and skeletal muscles – which perform more actively during periods of acute stress
- Redirect energy away from body activities such as growth, sex hormones, and digestion which are less critical for immediate survival.[11]

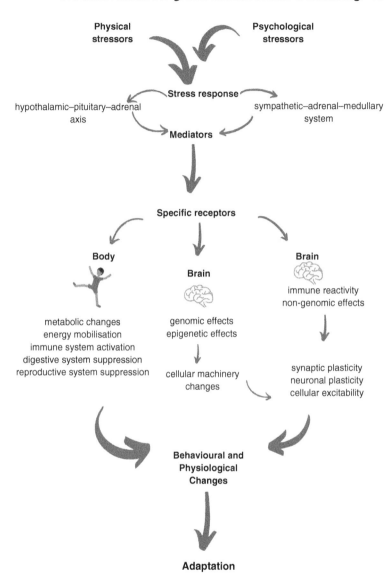

Figure 1.3 Stress response chemical cascade.[13]

The acute stress response directs this energy around the body to places where it is required, by the dilatation and contraction of blood vessels and by the cardiac output increasing via changes to the heart's stroke volume and rate (Figure 1.4).[12]

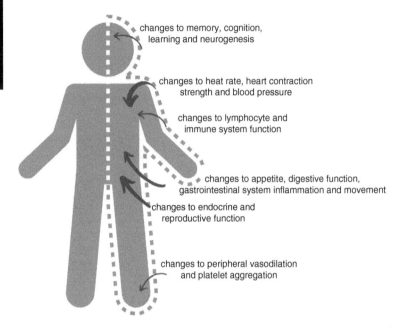

changes to memory, cognition, learning and neurogenesis

changes to heat rate, heart contraction strength and blood pressure

changes to lymphocyte and immune system function

changes to appetite, digestive function, gastrointestinal system inflammation and movement

changes to endocrine and reproductive function

changes to peripheral vasodilation and platelet aggregation

Figure 1.4   The stress response can impact on many different body systems.[14]

The sympathetic nervous system stimulates the adrenal medulla to produce catecholamine such as epinephrine. The hypothalamic-pituitary adrenocortical axis is also activated. Corticotropin releasing factor from the hypothalamus stimulates adrenocorticotropin from the pituitary gland. This stimulates cortisol secretion from the adrenal cortex.

Cortisol and catecholamines act to liberate energy sources by:

- Increasing glycogen conversion into glucose
- Increasing fat break down into energy sources such as glycerol and fatty acids.[11]

In young, healthy people, an acute stress response will more likely lead to a level of adaptation, rather than creating an actual health burden.[11,13] However, in less healthy or older people, it is more likely that repeated stress responses may be damaging to their health.[11]

Under chronic stress, this acute response may be repeatedly activated without resolving. Given the actions listed above of the acute stress response, continuous activation may lead to physical problems such as:

- Increased blood pressure
- Vascular hypertrophy
- Immune suppression

amongst other issues.

We know that prolonged exposure to stress is a risk factor for mental health conditions such as depression.[14] Prolonged stress can also exacerbate the symptoms of conditions such as bipolar and schizophrenia.[14]

Exposure to stress over long periods of time is likely to affect our efficiency at work. Evidence confirms that two out of three healthcare workers report significantly high levels of work stress, according to a UK workplace stress report.[15] It is clearly time to start doing something differently. Almost all of the healthcare workers – 95% – reported that the stress impacted tangibly on their lives, and almost half (47%) felt that their work-related stresses led them to suffer anxiety.

One in two health care workers in the UK reported that work-related stress has led to them suffering anxiety.

We use the pre-frontal cortex (PFC) region of our brain for many tasks that our daily jobs require us to successfully perform. The so-called 'higher executive functions' include planning, decision-making, and problem-solving. The PFC area is one of the most sensitive to stress.[14] We have good research evidence that our PFC is impaired under stress, leading to decreases in functions such as working memory.[16] Many of our required tasks as clinicians require the optimal functioning of our PFC, so it stands to reason that learning to manage our stress will help us be more effective in our work in various ways. When being stressed impairs our decision-making ability, this has the potential to impact negatively on patient outcomes – thus our work stress may lead to further work stress in a negative cycle.

Reduced functioning may also be linked to behaviours we fall back on during periods of stress, such as losing self-control, overeating, smoking, or excessive drinking.[14]

Problem factor: The diathesis-stress model

Numerous health conditions are categorised according to genes and their environmental interactions.[17] The diathesis-stress theory is the increased risk of a condition, such as depression, calculated by multiplying the impact of the genes by the environmental impact.[17]

'Diathesis' is a person's predisposition towards an illness, based on their specific set of biological factors.[17]

Much research supports an association that is significant between stressful life events and major depressive disorder.[17] Some of this even suggests that in more than half of the cases of depression, there is an instance of severe adversity.[18] The converse is also supported as true – that some of us will not present with cases of depression after severe life events. This evidence supports the idea that the symptom development is related to the complex interaction between how vulnerable and individual is – diathesis – and the stress that they are subject to.[17]

This model, which has been applied to many different psychopathologies, highlights that any periods of increased demand may be considered as stress. However, this may be a relevant way of viewing the impacts of crises and pandemics in the healthcare system, as these may be considered as serious life events for many clinicians. This reinforces the fact that during and after such events, additional support may be required, as we cover below.

We can do little about our genes, except perhaps to attempt to promote positive epigenetic changes in order to possibly affect their expression. We can, however, influence our environments – if not at the time of crisis or significant life event, then hopefully immediately after. Where we are unable to alter our external environment, we may potentially be able to at least change our internal – psychological – environment.

According to this model, there are certain points in life which act as serious life events. These may then, in turn, trigger mental health conditions in those of us who may, for many different reasons, have a genetic or biological vulnerability. We have little insight into predicting who has these vulnerabilities; however, with this information, we can aim to offer improved support to everyone in the wake of such events. This, in a healthcare context, may relate particularly to crises and pandemics which may act as such a trigger, as may other complex clinical cases.

Studies looking at the impact of COVID-19 on healthcare practitioners are also revealing the impact this crisis has had on us. One multi-centre study with 1,257 front-line staff in Wuhan, China found that healthcare staff who were involved in the care of patients with COVID-19 were associated with a greater risk of depression, insomnia, and anxiety symptoms.[19] Their levels of these symptoms were significantly higher than those of their colleagues in secondary roles, with men less likely than their female colleagues to report such symptoms.

Problem factor: Stigma

Mental health issues are subject to greater stigma than many other health conditions.[20] While there are an increasing number of conversations on mental health in the wider community, it is still a highly stigmatised area with regard to its impact on clinicians and other health professionals. There are a range of different resources for support with aspects of mental health for the general public, but there are significantly fewer specifically for clinicians. While these resources are relevant and supportive of anyone and everyone, the specific concerns of healthcare practitioners may at times need more specific support.

This stigma can create barriers to being able to seek access to care.[21] It can have different components– the emotional, the behavioural, the cognitive – as well as activities on different levels – the structural, the interpersonal, and the intrapersonal – that can be active all at once.[21]

> *Stigma may still act as a significant barrier to*
> *accessing mental health resources for clinicians.*

There is an extensive amount of research, some of which will be discussed in the coming pages, supporting the facts that clinicians are generally late to seek help for mental health conditions or to disclose their own mental health conditions. Despite treating patients with similar conditions, we are generally reluctant to seek help for ourselves.

By aiming to improve our own conversations that we have around our own mental health and wellbeing, we can also aim to improve the care that we can ultimately deliver to our patients.

Mental health conditions are also often subject to stereotypes. Stereotypes are useful in some areas of life, enabling us to make decisions based on patterns that we may have seen before – and so while these may not necessarily always be right, they may not necessarily always be harmful, either. However, with regards to mental health, stereotyping may lead to a generalised response pattern, rather than a customised one.[20] And given the obviously personal and widely differing natures of our mental health, it is clear that a generalised response based on a stereotype may not be the most helpful one. Stereotypes can also lead to characterisations of those affected as being completely defined by their condition, rather than recognising the ebbing and flowing nature of aspects of our mental – as with our physical – health.

Many factors may contribute to these feelings.[22] These factors, according to the Director of the Institute of Healthcare Policy and Innovation in the University of Michigan, USA, have the ability to 'lead to psychological symptoms'.[3] These include the stress of caring for colleagues who one moment have worked alongside of us, and the next moment are critically ill from COVID-19. Inevitably, some of these colleagues may pass away. The burden of caring for any patient who is acutely unwell is stressful – with this multiplied when there are multiple cases in rapid succession, with the potential to rapidly deteriorate. There is stress around the ability to provide adequate care, particularly when there are shortages in treatment devices such as ventilators, as well as concern about healthcare systems being inundated and pushed to breaking point. Given the changes in roles, stress can come from being allocated a different role in an area of clinical practice that we are less familiar with, as discussed. And finally, crucially, the lack of access to support services for managing these psychological symptoms is also a contributing factor.

The lack of suitable PPE can also cause significant stress. This stress may include a fear of contracting the virus through workplace, and a fear of transmitting it to family household members. These stresses led some clinicians to feeling that they needed to live away from their family during the pandemic, in turn bringing them additional stress through further straining their support network.

Moral injury, a term based initially on work within the military, may also occur when we have insufficient resources with which to care for critically unwell patients.[23] The term describes our feelings of psychological distress when our actions, or lack of actions, lead to us violating our ethical or moral code.[23] This can cause us to have negative thoughts about ourselves, and while it is not strictly a mental health condition, it may well affect our mental health.

Chapter 2 **Problem factors affecting healthcare practitioner mental health and wellbeing**

As discussed already, mental health and wellbeing are complex, with many aspects that are constantly in flux. The following problem factors are not specific only to clinicians and indeed may hold true for many other different occupations; however, they are particularly relevant in the healthcare industry.

Problem factor: Perceptions of invulnerability

As clinicians, we may be exposed to life and death situations on a daily basis. Our training may prepare us for these to a degree, although most of us can still vividly recall the first time we saw one of our patients pass away. How long we paused to reflect on their passing, as well as the transience of life and our own mortality, varies significantly – however most of us can recall, no matter how long ago it was, the first time we 'lost' someone.

In order to cope ourselves, we may develop a range of strategies.

From an external point of view, members of the community may wonder how we can cope with these pressures. Yet over time, many of us stop marvelling at the same thing. While this may, at times, be necessary in order to deliver good clinical care, as well as to maintain our own balance, occasionally recalling a bit of this wonder – and possibly a sense of critiquing how useful these strategies are – may be of benefit.

Research supports that this 'culture of invulnerability' may begin early, in training.[1] Within this is the idea that we are 'impervious to illness',[1] which clearly, we are not!

Conversations around the fact that mental health is a fluid aspect of our health, that at times it may be better, at times it may be worse and what we can do about it, may be helpful. It is also important to remember that we are not immune from mental health conditions, or any other conditions, nor are our colleagues. We are not immune to the very human feelings of loss. Being

How to Promote Wellbeing: Practical Steps for Healthcare Practitioners' Mental Health,
First Edition. Dr Rachel K. Thomas.

seen as invulnerable may obscure our own insight, as well as obscure our ability to see signs in our colleagues. Being able to notice and support vulnerabilities in our colleagues as well as ourselves is not a sign of failing or of weakness, but of the ability to learn. And having a higher threshold of sensitivity for these around times of crisis may help.

Even Biblical parables may be highlighting this fact – 'Physician, heal thyself' is a proverb from Luke.[2] Our ability to try to help others may be limited while ignoring or being blind to our own issues.

> *Mental health concerns, or needing support at times, are not signs of being a poor healthcare practitioner. They are signs of being human, and it is our humanity that ultimately makes us good at our profession.*

Suicide rates in doctors are higher than those in the general population, with increased prevalence in female doctors.[3] There is some evidence that the suicide rate for female doctors is approximately 3–4 times higher than the general population, and in the USA, that there is a 70% higher suicide and self-harm rate in USA physicians that are white and male when compared to members of other professions.[4] The suicide rate of female nurses is also increased.[5] Within the healthcare professions, other specialities such as dentistry, anaesthetics, and psychiatry are also at greater risk of suicide.[4]

Historically, philosophers such as Plato thought that a good physician was someone who had suffered from illness themselves, and not necessarily someone who was in the best of health.[6] Later, Jung coined the term 'wounded healers', writing that a physician who was wounded could heal most effectively.[7]

Later ideas, such as those of psychiatrist Viktor Frankl, explored suffering as a fundamental part of the human experience. His book was based on his time in Nazi concentration camps. Frankl considered that suffering must have meaning, if we assume that life has meaning, and given that suffering is part of life.[8]

We may have a greater sense of solidarity and understanding with our patients, if we consider that many of us may actually even be 'wounded healers' ourselves.[6] We may realise that being able to acknowledge our own challenges, which could even have influenced our decision to become a clinician, is invaluable.

Problem factor: Presenteeism

In some occupations, absenteeism may be used as a proxy for staff wellbeing. How often people take sick days may be used to see how well the organisation is functioning as regards supporting the mental and physical health of its employees.

Presenteeism, by contrast, is when we go to work despite having an illness which may prevent our complete functioning while there.[9] We, as healthcare practitioners, may often deny ourselves the right to take time off work when feeling unwell, either mentally or physically. This may then lead to a knock-on effect of poorer outcomes, both for ourselves, our patients, and our colleagues, and may result in actually increasing stress.

Research into the costs of absenteeism and presenteeism reveals some surprising results. The cost of presenteeism is more than the cost of absenteeism. In one study, the cost of presenteeism was $3,055 per person per year, significantly more than the $520 per person per year of absenteeism.[10] Furthermore, it found that one of the total cost burdens that was the highest was associated with mental health conditions.[10]

It may be interesting to reflect on whether, in the last year, we feel we have gone to work feeling impaired, mentally or physically, to the point of being unfit. Commit to ticking one option, after reflecting on last year:

☐ Yes
☐ No

If we have ticked 'yes', we are certainly not alone. Many of us involved in healthcare feel obliged to work despite knowing we are sick. It may seem that the trade-off between staying home, versus going to work to help our patients and colleagues, is an easy and justifiable decision to make. But when we start to consider the cost of potentially infecting our patients and affecting their outcomes, infecting our colleagues and their ability to work, and the costs that are associated with all of this, the decision becomes less clear. Furthermore, we may be delaying our own ability to heal, thus drawing out the process even longer.

If we have ever felt under pressure to come to work when we are sick, then we are most certainly not alone. One study reported that 64% of allied health professionals, nurses, and aides, and 83% of medical practitioners, did not take sick leave with 'influenza-like illnesses'.[11] During the recent pandemic, there was clearer guidance on staying at home for those with symptoms of the infection. Similarly, there tends to be clearer guidance on staying home for a specific period, until symptoms have cleared, during repeated outbreaks of norovirus.

Presenteeism can cause a range of negative impacts. We are less able to carry out our work as efficiently, safely, and effectively as usual, and thus can increase our colleagues' workloads as they 'pick up the slack'. We also risk transmitting infectious disease to a patient population which is, by definition, already more vulnerable. And while due to budgets and staffing limitations this may remain a factor at least in the short term, it is still worth consideration. This idea of presenteeism generally extends beyond a lack of insight into our own illness or need for time off. There are usually more complex factors at play; however, it may also feed into being a barrier to accessing help.[1] These factors may include us feeling that we are letting our colleagues down if we take time off work.

The pressures to attend work when we are unwell can seem great, even though we may be aware that we are delaying our own healing or exacerbating our own illness, as well as being a risk to our patients. When considering that a patient may not be reviewed or treated because we chose to stay at home in bed and drink tea, staying home is generally not a choice we make. Knowing that our co-workers will have to do more work to cover us, in areas where there is inadequate staffing, may further weigh into our decision-making process. Our sense of personal responsibility to our patients and co-workers needs to be weighed against our responsibility towards ourselves and a recognition that if we are attending work in order to help, we may actually be a danger to both our colleagues and patients through illness transmission, poorer care, and a longer disease cycle for ourselves – and so, ultimately, who are we even actually helping?

In the same vein as in an aeroplane emergency, we should put on our own oxygen mask first before helping others; at times taking a sick day when we are unwell is the best course of action.

Greater organisational change may be required in order to help fight aspects of presenteeism. A study found that providing as little as three paid sick days without the requirement of a medical certificate led to less presenteeism (defined as working while sick) without more sick days being taken.[12] Furthermore, having defined 'back-to-work' rules such as a longer period before an ill worker can return for certain conditions may actually paradoxically lead to a decrease in the total number of sick days taken on an institutional level, due to reducing the number of sick staff members.[13] During COVID-19, clear rules around staying home if we were displaying any symptoms of the disease meant that we were clear on when we could come to work. These guidelines were spelled out for the nation to help limit the spread of the virus, too. In doing so, there was decreased ambiguity – and decreased guilt – about when it was time to stay home.

In the section on organisational protective factors discussed in greater detail below, the conversation around presenteeism needs consideration from staffing and rota departments. Potential solutions are complicated, and as far-reaching as ensuring the recruitment of adequate numbers of clinicians.

Problem factor: Perceptions of hierarchy

Historically, relatively paternalistic attitudes within medicine, surgery, and general healthcare may have added to restricted feelings on speaking about how we are feeling. In the past, this hierarchy facilitated the 'top' to speak, while 'lower down' listened. The consultant declared and the juniors took notes. And so some clinicians may feel that their freedom of expression is influenced - and limited - by this perception of hierarchy.

Inequality amongst feeling able to express concerns – be they about our work environment, how we feel, or about our colleagues – may have been compounded by a lack of safe reporting mechanisms.

When clinicians feel disempowered to voice how they are feeling, there are multiple significant impacts. Not only can it compound the stresses and pressures we are under by removing a coping mechanism – discussion – from us; it also serves to deprive the organisation of potentially powerful and restorative new ideas which could provide solutions for current and future colleagues.

A study into the wellbeing of nurses concluded that 'stress resulting from conflicts with supervisors was independently associated with mental health'.[14] Some of this stress may have been related to this sense of hierarchy.

While the rigidity of the hierarchy in medicine and surgery is certainly shifting, there are still remnants that affect how freely we feel we can express ourselves with those who are our seniors – despite them potentially being best placed to help us. In not being able to express how we are feeling, we are actually deprived of one of our best supports.

A culture of a strict hierarchy may be linked to bullying.

Linked to this may be a culture of bullying. Research supports that the risk of workplace bullying amongst health care practitioners may be as high as twice that of people employed by the government, at around 8% in some areas.[15] Research supports that this may be higher in the UK, with one study of nearly 3,000 NHS workers indicating that over 40% of staff had witnessed bullying, and 20% of staff had been subject to it, in the six months prior.[16] This negatively affected how satisfied staff were with their job, increased their desire and intention to leave, and was associated with decreased psychological health. This study reported that there were several barriers to reporting bullying, which included a view that the bullying would not change and how the case would be managed. It was also linked to the seniority of the bully – many of whom were most commonly managers.

Problem factor: Burnout

Burnout is a problem that is, of course, not specific to clinicians. It can affect any of us, irrespective of how and where we work. We discuss burnout here because its emergence has become a significant issue in the healthcare community.

The term 'burnout' is being used more and more frequently when we, as clinicians, discuss our careers. It is often used loosely, referring to people who have been working too hard, for too long, and are simply unable to sustain it. Like a flame that has used up all the available oxygen and resources to stay alight, it has simply gone out.

> *'Burnout is reflected in pathological emotional depletion and maladaptive detachment that is a secondary result of exposure to prolonged occupational stress.'* [17]

Burnout has recently been included as a classification in the International Classification of Diseases (ICD-11) as an occupational phenomenon.[18] The previous classification, ICD-10, included burnout, but in ICD-11, the recent revision, the definition is more detailed. Burnout is not classified as a 'medical condition' but is included as a factor which impacts health status negatively and prompts people to contact health services.

According to ICD-11, burnout is a syndrome which results from unsuccessfully managed chronic workplace stress. The definition is specific to workplace and occupational stress and is not applicable to other life areas.[19]

Burnout has three defining characteristics:

- *'Feelings of energy depletion or exhaustion*
- *Increased mental distance from one's job, or feelings of negativism or cynicism related to one's job*
- *Reduced professional efficacy.'*[19]

The WHO is devising evidence-based guidelines to promote workplace mental wellbeing. The decision to include burnout as an issue that impacts on our health, and to have burnout included in the revised ICD-11, highlights the significance of burnout in the workplace.

The president of the World Medical Association, Dr Leonid Eidelman stated:

> *'For too long burnout among physicians has been largely ignored. Emotionally exhausted physicians are a danger to patients and a danger to themselves. The cost in terms of human lives and money is appalling.'*[20]

Burnout was first defined in 1974 by Freudenberger as the type of emotional exhaustion that is experienced by public service workers.[21] He saw burnout as linked to something that occurred when there was a failure to obtain the results and rewards expected from a professional relationship.

This definition was further expanded by Maslach and Jackson in 1986 into a multidimensional construct.[22] In Maslach's definition, professional relationships were particularly those in human service professions, including not only healthcare workers but also police, lawyers, teachers, and more. This has been shaped into an inventory, called the Maslach Burnout Inventory (MBI), which can be used to identify and measure our risk of burnout. The MBI describes a more psychological syndrome and focuses on three dimensions in the definition: personal accomplishment, depersonalisation and emotional exhaustion.

According to this expanded definition, personal accomplishment relates to feelings of being successful, or competent, and achieving goals at work. Someone is at higher risk of burnout if their feelings relate to a decrease in this area, including feelings such as inadequacy and incompetence.

Depersonalisation relates to a decreased connection with patients, potentially even treating them more as objects than as people, and often including negative attitudes towards them. It may also include starting to feel cynical towards them. An increase in this area puts someone at a higher risk of burnout on the inventory, as exemplified by feeling increasingly impersonal towards the people that we are caring for. Emotional exhaustion relates to feeling overextended emotionally, perhaps to the point of emptiness and a feeling that there is 'nothing left' to be given. It may also be coupled with feelings such as tiredness. An increase in this area, feeling increasingly exhausted or overextended emotionally, may be linked to a higher risk of burnout on the inventory.

A 2019 study by the British Medical Association of over 4,300 medical students and doctors found that:

- 40% of respondents were experiencing burnout, anxiety, depression, emotional distress, stress, or mental health conditions that impacted on their study, work, and/or training
- 27% of respondents had at some point in their life received a mental health condition diagnosis
- 7% of respondents received a mental health diagnosis in the last year.[23]

Concerningly, 80% – the majority of the respondents – were at either very high risk or high risk of burnout (Figure 2.1) – with those at the highest risk being junior doctors. Also, 90% of GP partners were also in this very high risk, or high risk, of burnout category.

Given the high levels of stress that we experience in our roles, doctors are considered particularly susceptible to burnout [24] Those working at the front line, or at the first point of care, may have the highest risk of burnout [25] A study in rural British Columbia had sobering results:

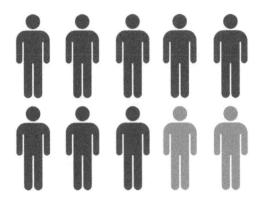

Figure 2.1   Around 8 in 10 respondents were at high or very high risk of burnout.[23]

- 44% had low to moderate feelings with regards to Personal Accomplishment
- 61% had severe to moderate feelings with regards to Depersonalisation
- 80% had severe to moderate Emotional Exhaustion.[26]

The results of other studies are not dissimilar, with about one third of UK doctors having a high burnout score on the MBI in at least one area [27]

A study of 8,000 surgeons showed links between burnout and medical errors. Using a depersonalisation scale with increments from 0–33, a one-point increase was associated with an increased error reporting likelihood of 11%. Using an emotional exhaustion scale with increments from 0–54, an increase of one-point was associated with an increased error reporting likelihood of 5%. Burnout was shown to be an independent predictor of major medical error reporting.[28]

And the impact and implications of this are far-reaching. They go well beyond impacting merely on our own mental health or career progression, although there is significant evidence to support links with an increased risk of:

- Anxiety
- Depression
- Disturbed sleep and fatigue
- Misusing alcohol and drugs – prescription and/or illicit
- Dysfunction in relationships such as marriage
- Early retirement
- Suicide.

Evidence supports that burnout can significantly impact patient outcomes, too. Studies show that burnout is related to decreases in cognitive control and execution functioning, including areas such as reasoning, problem solving, planning, working memory, and execution.[29] Burnout has been linked to a range of detrimental impacts on practice, such as:

- Increased hostility towards patients
- Greater risk of poor decision-making
- Increased rate of medical errors
- Increased difficulty in relationship maintenance with colleagues and co-workers.

Given the multiple negative potential impacts on care and outcomes, we should cultivate ways in which to protect ourselves from burnout – not only for our own sakes, but for those of our patients and colleagues too.

A study of 130 critical care unit clinicians looked at how burnout related to healthcare-associated infections (Figure 2.2).[30] It concluded that decreasing rates of burnout was a useful strategy in decreasing infections – thus improving not only the clinicians' wellbeing but patient care, too. It stated that burnout was especially a problem for these clinicians due to their high responsibilities, high patient acuity, and degrees of chronic stress they were under. It found that 'high work demands' lead to emotional exhaustion and cynicism. This in turn affected how teams communicated, which affected

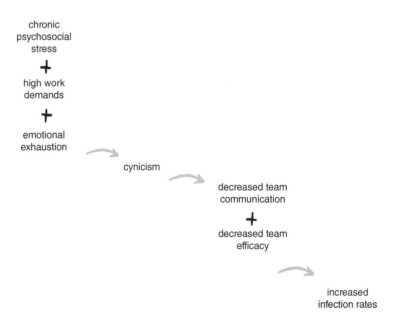

Figure 2.2 Possible links between stress and infection rates.[30]

how effective a team was. This 'team efficacy' then affected rates of health-care-associated infection.[30]

Another study concluded that a promising strategy to help infection control in acute care is to reduce burnout.[31] In this study, more than a third of the nurses involved reported that their job-related burnout levels were high. Based on this research, it was concluded that if the average of 30% of nurses with high burnout could be reduced to 10%, 4,160 infections could be prevented, and at a saving of over $40 million.[31]

Overall, burnout can lead to poorer quality of care, decreased patient safety, and decreased patient satisfaction. A decrease in patient satisfaction is strongly linked with an increase in the number of complaints and an increase in medicolegal or dentolegal risk – all of which can further act to increase stresses and nudge us towards burnout.

The extent, and possibly the likelihood of burnout may depend upon different factors, such as:

- Speciality
- Stage in career
- Clinical environments and practice settings
- Changes to the work environment.

While there are a range of protective factors we can possess, and skills that we can learn, these are often not covered or taught until we are already feeling the effects of excessive stress levels or burnout ourselves.

As many of us may recall from exams, trying to learn new skills when stressed can be difficult! We may find that we need new wellbeing skills most at a time when we may feel the least capable of learning them. Therefore, these are skills we should start trying to learn – if not master – well before needing them.

In a study of dentists, almost 10% had burnout.[32] Other research suggests that burnout rates may be up to 75% in groups such as resident doctors and is associated with negative attitudes towards patient care.[33] This study even concluded that resident doctors should have burnout interventions, to address burnout and its negative impacts on the care of patients. It found that the residents who had burnout were at a greater likelihood of behaviours that were associated with poorer clinical care. These included not fully answering questions, not fully discussing the available treatment options, making medication errors, making treatment errors, ignoring the personal impact of an illness, ignoring the social impact of an illness, the discharge of patients in order to make the healthcare service easier to manage, and then ultimately having a feeling of guilt about a patient's treatment. Indeed, high levels of burnout in clinicians has been supported by research in many different areas of the world (Figure 2.3).

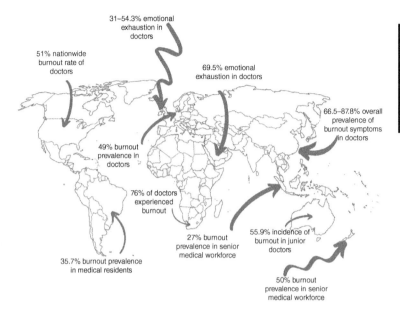

31–54.3% emotional exhaustion in doctors

51% nationwide burnout rate of doctors

69.5% emotional exhaustion in doctors

66.5–87.8% overall prevalence of burnout symptoms in doctors

49% burnout prevalence in doctors

76% of doctors experienced burnout

27% burnout prevalence in senior medical workforce

55.9% incidence of burnout in junior doctors

35.7% burnout prevalence in medical residents

50% burnout prevalence in senior medical workforce

Chapter 2

Figure 2.3 High levels of burnout in clinicians has been supported by research in many different areas of the world.[34, 35, 36, 37, 38, 39, 40, 41, 42, 43]

The emotional cost of our workloads as clinicians is not often openly discussed. Evidence shows that a broad range of emotions are felt during the course of healthcare-related interactions, and that the emotional needs of a patient are often responded to with our own emotions.[44] Commonly, these emotions may include feeling like we have failed if a patient deteriorates, feeling that we are powerless when facing certain illnesses, feeling that we need to somehow rescue our patients, or even feeling that we need to disengage from, and avoid connection with, our patients in order to not feel these feelings.

While this is normal, it is also important to realise that we should try to both identify and control these emotions in order to deliver optimal patient care, as well as to promote our own wellbeing. Without doing so, unexamined emotions can lead to impacts such as poorer clinical judgement, disengagement, and ultimately burnout.

While repeated cycles of emotions related to patients can contribute to burnout, other factors inherent in the healthcare infrastructure also play a significant role. These environments are becoming increasingly litigious.[45] There are often additional requirements from middle management and bureaucracy. It is not uncommon for one change to come in effect, and then as soon as we have adjusted to it, for there to be yet another iteration added to then adjust to.

A study by the Medical Protection Society in the UK revealed that 57% of doctors felt that they were not able to take breaks even if these were short, and 68% said it was not usual to get a rest period during a shift; and 80% of nurses reported not being able to get a single drink for their whole shift, with this happening weekly for more than half of them.[46] Thus, advice for us to take breaks is difficult to both give and receive while the organisations that we work within are contributing to this type of feeling. We are stretched by staffing issues and spread across changing rotas. We may find that the administrative or paperwork-based aspects of our roles are increasing, leaving less time for patient and clinical interactions. As already discussed, a doctor falling ill or leaving the rota often leads to further stretching of those that remain. Even the process of obtaining leave for important occasions can be difficult.

There are always additional changes to the content of what we must know, with guidelines and advances constantly evolving [47] It is our responsibility to maintain our professional standards in relation to this; however, this can be an additional source of pressure and stress. This is further compounded by the fact that, at times, we may find ourselves in roles that are, in the purest sense, beyond what we trained for. This is particularly the case when there are efforts to rapidly expand the capabilities of the healthcare system, as with the COVID-19 pandemic.

Constantly evolving guidelines, and the demands around staying compliant with these, can lead to an increase in clinician stress.

There is also an inherent stress from the fact that our healthcare resources are finite. Again, this was sharply highlighted in the recent pandemic. There are pressures associated with the allocation of these finite resources, and how just or unjust this allocation may be.

Problem factor: Compassion fatigue

Compassion fatigue has been defined in several ways. One of these is 'stress resulting from exposure to a traumatised individual'.[48] It is essentially when cumulative aspects of burnout meet with traumatic stresses, leading to decreased ability to cope with day-to-day environments and feeling mentally and physically exhausted.[48] Given the daily exposure that we, as clinicians, may have to such events, we are at a greater susceptibility to compassion fatigue. Evidence supports that it impacts on many aspects – both professional and personal. These include our:

- Patient care
- Colleague relationships
- Mental health.[48]

Compassion fatigue presents in a range of ways. Some of these include:

- Feeling exhausted
- Feeling angry or irritable
- Negative coping behaviours such as drinking excessively
- Increased rates of absenteeism
- Decreased decision-making capacity at work
- Decreased feelings of empathy and sympathy
- Decreased feelings of enjoyment at work.[48]

Compassion fatigue may be related to burnout, but is not necessarily the same thing – however, both are related to 'outcomes of exposure'.[49] Compassion fatigue is '*the progressive and cumulative outcome of prolonged, continuous, and intense contact with patients, self-utilisation, and exposure to multidimensional stress leading to a compassion discomfort that exceeds a nurse's endurance levels*'.[50] The energy required to maintain compassion may be beyond restoration, leading to progressive changes in many areas, including:

- Intellectual
- Spiritual
- Social
- Physical
- Emotional.[50]

It is usually people in carer roles who experience compassion fatigue. As a part of this, they may feel their levels of 'caring' decrease – which can lead to a range of complicated feelings, including a confusing sense of 'lost identity'. Compassion fatigue has symptoms and signs similar to those present in post-traumatic stress disorder (PTSD).[51] These include re-running the experience mentally, efforts to avoid situations, and feeling hyper-aroused.[51]

In contrast, burnout relates more to negative attitudes, behaviours, and responses caused by job strain, leading to feelings such as feeling powerless, frustrated, and unable to meet the goals required at work.[50]

Moral distress, where we feel we are not able to act in a way that aligns with our values due to external reasons beyond our control, can lead not only to lower job satisfaction and to leaving the profession, but also to reacting aggressively to situations.[51]

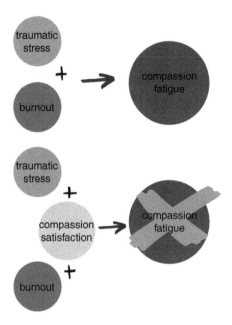

Figure 2.4　Compassion fatigue as conceptually linked to stress, burnout, and compassion satisfaction.[52]

It is therefore perhaps unsurprising that burnout and traumatic stress may both contribute to feelings of compassion fatigue (Figure 2.4).

The above diagram outlines how burnout and traumatic stress lead to compassion fatigue, particularly without the protective factor of compassion satisfaction. Burnout is depicted as a type of survival strategy, linked to when we are unable to achieve our goal and have an '*assertiveness–goal achievement response*'.[48] When we aren't able to achieve whatever that particular goal may be – in this setting, most likely related to patient outcomes or welfare – there is '*frustration, a sense of loss of control, increased wilful efforts, and diminishing morale*'.[53] By contrast, traumatic stress relates to a '*rescue–caretaking response*', activated when we are not able to rescue someone – presumably a patient – from distress.[53] Compassion satisfaction can be seen as a potentially mitigating or protective factor, related to the positive results of working in this area, as we will discuss more fully later.

Research supports that both burnout and compassion fatigue lead to a range of negative consequences in areas including:

- Practitioner job-related satisfaction
- Practitioner wellbeing
- Patient outcomes
- Patient healthcare satisfaction.[50]

Crucially, compassion fatigue may also have an impact on willingness to continue in healthcare professions, as well as on job turn-over.[50]

Problem factor: Perfectionistic personality traits

There are high rates of perfectionism and its traits in many high achievers, including clinicians.[54] While it is undoubtedly important to maintain high quality clinical care, perfectionism can contribute to job stress and ultimately burnout.

Practising effectively in healthcare means we often need to balance opposing aspects. We need to be able to connect empathetically with our patients. However, we also need to preserve an appropriate element of detachment in order to provide appropriate clinical care. Being consumed by emotion would obscure clear and rational thought, critical for decision-making. Detachment is also needed to help us switch our focus from one patient to the following one in the next bed or consultation, giving them optimum care too. On a human level, if we are too attached to the suffering associated with disease, our own emotional survival is jeopardised.

Furthermore, if we have perfectionistic traits, this may increase often already high levels of criticism of ourselves and our work. While a healthy dose of self-criticism and thorough thought can improve clinical care, it becomes obsessional if excessive, and is linked to higher rates of depression.

Unchecked perfectionism leads us to never feeling as though we have done our job well enough. Any mistakes we perceive lead us to becoming highly self-critical, even to losing confidence in our own abilities. Learning to ensure that we continue to set ourselves high standards, and yet let these become a little relaxed if the situation demands it, helps to balance any perfectionism.

Therapists have a variety of scales with which to determine perfectionistic traits. However, a generalised, light-hearted and non-scientific screen developed by Flett highlights some unhealthy perfectionistic traits.

'Top Ten Signs Your a Perfectionist

1. *You cannot stop thinking about a mistake you made.*
2. *You are intensely competitive and can't stand doing worse than others.*
3. *You either want to do something 'just right' or not at all.*
4. *You demand perfection from other people.*
5. *You will not ask for help if asking can be perceived as a flaw or weakness.*
6. *You will persist at a task long after other people have quit.*
7. *You are a faultfinder who must correct other people when they are wrong.*
8. *You are highly aware of other people's demands and expectations.*

9. *You are very self-conscious about making mistakes in front of other people.*
10. *You noticed the error in the title of this list.'*[55]

Psychological distress has been found to strongly correlate with perfectionism in studies with pharmacy, medical, nursing, and dental students.[56] Perfectionistic tendencies lead us into taking on additional responsibilities in efforts to ensure work is done 'perfectly'. This may result in us becoming more tired and drained than if we had delegated effectively.

Problem factor: Lack of recovery behaviours

Most careers inevitably have at least some periods of high stress. For various reasons, different careers are encouraged to handle these periods in different ways.

Professional athletes have periods of exceptionally high stress as a common part of their career. The stresses they may be under during these times are both mental and physical. It is commonly accepted that a professional athlete, in order to succeed, pays attention to optimising both the mental and physical aspects of their performance, and their recovery.

Athletes realise that in order to function at the 'top of their game', they need to ensure that they have not only adequate training, but also adequate rest and recovery. As part of their training, they may have a team that includes a:

- Nutritionist
- Physiotherapist
- Psychologist
- Coach
- Adviser.

Athletes have off-season training, as well as on-season. In their on-season training, there may be cycles of training to build strength, skill, and endurance and to then promote recovery.

While a career as a clinician is undoubtedly different from an athlete's, it is useful for anyone working in a high-stress career to look at the structure of the athlete's career and the recovery behaviours that they utilise.

These recovery behaviours include aspects such as:

- Relaxation techniques
- Visualisation techniques
- Nutrition support
- Adequate sleep
- Periods of decreased demand
- Alternative training activities.

Being able to move between focused, performance promoting behaviours and the effective use of recovery behaviours enables an athlete to optimise not only their performance but also their career duration.

· There is a balance between how many recovery behaviours we can implement independently and how many require institutional support. Obviously, being able to have both these facets leads to increased recovery and support. Realistically, making changes to those of our behaviours that are under our own control is a simpler starting point than trying to change those of our behaviours that depend on support from our work environment.

Problem factor: Sleep cycle derangement and sleep deprivation

There is an increasing body of research on the importance of sleep. This activity that we spend about a third of our life doing is currently a source of much discussion, with evidence supporting its key role in areas such as memory formation and even dementia.

As clinicians, our sleep will at times be sacrificed as an expected part of our work. It's no small comfort to know that approximately 20% of us in Europe and America work shifts in the night, with shift work defined as any schedule expanding past the 9am to 5pm working day. Up to 5% of these workers may still have their sleep affected up to one month after the work schedule.[57] This impact depends on other factors such as how long the schedule impacts on the sleep, the time frame between night shifts, and how predictable the schedule is. These relationships are multifactorial and complex, with personal factors also playing a role in how well an individual can cope with night shifts.

For many clinicians, night shifts are unavoidable since they are a key component of any effectively running hospital with inpatients. Without overnight care, there is not adequate continuing care for inpatients. While it may not be necessary to be awake all night, or even to sleep onsite, someone, somewhere has their sleep affected when there are inpatients. Night shifts are one of the most common reasons for disturbed sleep patterns and circadian rhythm disruption. Hence there is an organisational and systemic feature, which is a stress on our wellbeing, that is built into the healthcare system. So, given that this is inevitable, how can we best manage these stresses and their impact on us?

We know that shift work is linked to a range of issues. A study of clinicians looked specifically at whether or not night shifts had negative impacts on areas of physical and mental health.[58] The areas studied included:

- Cardiovascular symptoms
- Psychological symptoms

- Fatigue symptoms
- Sleep quality and quantity
- Job satisfaction.

The study found that night shifts significantly negatively impacted on these aspects. Results showed a significantly lower mean score in various areas, when compared to workers on the day shift. The study concluded that clinicians on a rotating night schedule were at higher risk of undesirable health effects, compared to those on day shift. It also concluded that those on night shift were at greater risk of job dissatisfaction. Other research concludes that decreases in job satisfaction are strongly associated with increases in job stress.[59] Therefore, job satisfaction may be responsive to stress management interventions. This further elevates the importance of increasing resilience and other mechanisms that buffer against the effects of stress.

Tiredness can lead to greater impairment in concentration and performance at these times and, in turn, negatively impact on patient outcomes. Handovers at the end of a night shift – and particularly if done in a rushed or inadequate fashion due to tiredness – can continue to impact on patient care during the following day.

On a particularly busy night shift, Mrs J.E. in Bed 3 and Mr E.K. in Bed 4 both had chest pain. Investigation results were not back at the end of the shift. If we are tired, we may rush through the handover, and it may not be clear to the day team that there are two separate sets of results needing follow-up, significantly affecting patient care the following day.

The impacts of night shifts extend beyond the hospital walls, too. There is a significant increase in the risk of having an accident while driving home at the conclusion of a shift, through factors such as impaired concentration or falling asleep at the wheel.

Obviously also the stress from our roles in the daytime hours negatively impacts on our ability to sleep. Sleep-promoting activities, such as exercise and regular waking hours, can be difficult to incorporate into our lifestyle. However, as we will discuss, certain strategies may be able to help with this.

Chapter 3 **Problem and protective factors affecting patients' mental health and wellbeing**

The aim of this book is to highlight aspects affecting the mental health and wellbeing of us, clinicians. However, a motivating reason for many of us doing our job is the desire to help people. This is basically providing our patients with the best outcomes possible. While our focus in this book is on the problems and solutions concerning clinician mental health and wellbeing, it would be remiss to not include, at least briefly, factors to be considered that relate to patient mental health and wellbeing, also. Positive outcomes related to patient mental health and wellbeing also lead to positive outcomes for clinicians, and the development of a 'virtuous circle' (Figure 3.1).

While we may feel our job is already too busy to spend time considering the mental health and wellbeing factors in our patients, we should remember how important these factors are. Information on both problem and protective factors relating to the mental health and wellbeing of the patients is included together here in this section, before we move on to examine the protective factors for our own mental health and wellbeing in more detail in the following chapters.

Factor to consider: The interlinkage of mental and physical health

There is a growing amount of evidence supporting the interconnectedness between our physical and mental health. For instance, evidence shows that depression is not only more common in patients who have cardiac events, it is also a risk factor, impacting on both mortality and morbidity, and independent of other risk factors.[1] One study found that depressive symptoms were a greater risk for heart disease than passive smoking was (1.64 versus 1.25, respectively).[2]

Similarly, research shows that patients with other conditions such as chronic pain, as well as depression, have health outcomes that are poorer

How to Promote Wellbeing: Practical Steps for Healthcare Practitioners' Mental Health,
First Edition. Dr Rachel K. Thomas.
© 2021 Dr Rachel K. Thomas. Published 2021 by John Wiley & Sons Ltd.

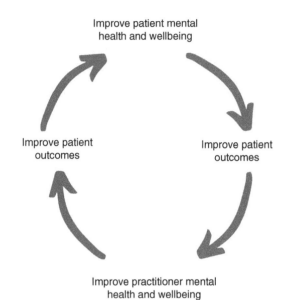

Improve patient mental
health and wellbeing

Improve patient
outcomes

Improve patient
outcomes

Improve practitioner mental
health and wellbeing

Figure 3.1 A virtuous cycle indicating how improving mental health can improve patient outcomes.

than patients who have only chronic pain, and that treating the depression helps decrease their pain.[3]

There are similar results for other areas, too, such as lung disease. Depression is associated with a decrease in quality of life and functional performance, and an increase in shortness of breath in patients with Chronic Obstructive Pulmonary disease (COPD), and therefore treating depression may be important clinically for these patients.[4]

Given the connection between mental and physical health, we can improve patient outcomes by screening for, and considering, mental health aspects in them, too. Even though this may not be an area of our expertise, or even of our interest, our goal in providing optimal patient care means that its consideration may be necessary. Traditionally, medicine is viewed as systems. We start early in our training as 'generalists' and over time, progressively 'specialise'. Since there is increasing evidence that mental health and wellbeing impacts on physical health, it is relevant for us to consider aspects of our patients' mental health and wellbeing in relation to their physical health in a less 'systems-based' manner.

Considering our patients' mental health and wellbeing may improve their clinical outcomes for physical conditions.

It is worthwhile further examining the link between depression and its increased occurrence in patients with cardiovascular disease.[1] Depression

Table 3.1   The Patient Health Questionnaire (PHQ-2).[5]

Over the last two weeks, how often have you been bothered by any of the following problems?	Not at all	Several days	More than half of the days	Nearly every day
Little interest or pleasure in doing things?	0	1	2	3
Feeling down, depressed or hopeless?	0	1	2	3

is also positively associated with repeated cardiac events, quality of life, and even mortality.[1] Various mechanisms have been proposed to elicit the link between depression and cardiovascular disease – from inflammation to decreased involvement in health-promoting activities. The American Heart Association recommends that cardiac patients are screened routinely for depression with screening tools such as the Patient Health Questionnaire (two- or nine-item versions PHQ-2 or PHQ-9). The PHQ-2 is the first two questions on the PHQ-9, and may be useful for preliminary screening of patients (Table 3.1).

The National Institute for Health and Care Excellence (NICE), an independent organisation, produces evidence-based guidelines for clinical practice, evaluating medications and procedures. NICE guidance for screening patients at risk of depression recommends two short questions:

- 'During the last month have you often been feeling down, depressed, or hopeless?
- During the last month have you often been bothered by having little interest or pleasure in doing things?'.[5]

A patient responding 'yes' to at least one of these questions is highly specific for depression, but with low sensitivity ((0.95, 95% CI 0.91 to 0.97) and (0.66, 95% CI 0.55 to 0.76) respectively).[5] If this is positive, other tools like the Patient Health Questionnaire 9 (PHQ-9) can then be used.[6] For anxiety, the Generalised Anxiety Disorder Questionnaire (GAD-7) consisting of seven questions may be useful.

Remember that we may often be seeing patients at difficult times in their life. They may feel scared of the potential implications of their condition, as well as the process of hospitalisation. It is an unfamiliar setting where they are basically in the hands of someone else for most things they would normally do themselves. Even their meals are delivered differently, with possibly different foods and at different times, all of which they may have little control over. If we keep this in mind, it may help our patient interactions. Particularly during the recent pandemic, this fear of being hospitalised was exacerbated by seeing clinicians dressed in PPE, and by concerns over catching the virus while actually in hospital. Hospital admissions even decreased as a reflection of patients not presenting due to concern over becoming infected while in hospital.

The importance of non-verbal communication is widely recognised and is discussed more fully later on. Our facial expressions are an important part of how we communicate, and they are important in building rapport and expressing empathy. To have simple gestures such as smiles obscured by masks, and the masks also hindering verbal communication, would add to the uncertainty – and potentially stress – around hospital interactions. And empathy is supported in evidence as being greatly significant in patient outcomes.[7]

Mental symptoms sometimes exacerbate, and sometimes *obscure*, physical symptoms in patients. Research suggests that at least 10% of symptoms which appear to be psychological actually have physical conditions underlying them.[8] And physical health issues may increase mental health ones. There is a significant correlation between the symptoms of depression and all-cause mortality.[9] Depression also correlates with higher natural deaths.[9]

Factor to consider: Sleep

In a perfect world, hospitals would be places where our patients were safely nurtured, with all aspects of their health and wellbeing optimised in order to support therapies, and their bodies, fighting off infection, illness, or injury. The reality, of course, is somewhat more dystopian. To put it bluntly, hospital admissions may have a negative impact on aspects of lifestyle which could, instead, have been more supportive for patients.

There is a significant and growing body of research on the importance of sleep. It is critical for a range of functions, including healing. It is thought that it may have a role in immunological memory formation.[10] For instance, research supports that sleeping the night after a vaccination produced a 'strong and persistent increase in the number of antigen-specific T cells and antibody titres'.[10] Models suggest that when sleep is fragmented, it may cause delays in wound healing.[11]

Wards can still be awash with noise and light during the sleep hours. Many monitors have bright blue light displays and are usually placed close to each patient bed. Nocturnal administration of medications and other healthcare interventions are commonplace. Unsurprisingly, hospitalisation is often an additionally stressful time for patients. They are in a foreign environment, understandably concerned about what will happen to them and whether they will recover. All of these, and other, factors, accumulate and often translate into poor sleep quantity and quality for the inpatient, It is not uncommon for their sleep to finally arrive just as we are appearing on our ward rounds.

There is a considerable amount of evidence around the impact of blue light on sleep.[12] The impact varies according to the individual, as well as to factors such as the quantity, duration of exposure, and luminosity. However, many bedside monitors and observation machines in hospital have brightly lit interfaces. The staff areas in wards are also usually brightly lit. While there is always a trade-off of the visibility of patients for safety reasons, versus darkness for them to sleep, it is worth considering making small improvements.

Small considerations like turning the bright light from observation trolleys away from the patient's direct line of sight when they are trying to sleep may help, as long as this is not interfering with how clinicians can see them. In some suitable cases, earplugs or eye masks may be of benefit to patients, and these could be brought in by relatives or friends, and are even offered by some hospitals.

Efforts to draw curtains to decrease ambient light at the same time each day, in order to facilitate a bedtime routine for patients may help – especially during summer months. And while we are all busy in meeting the expectations and demands of our own jobs, at least trying to factor in points such as these may help patients feel more cared for, as well as potentially improving their outcomes.

Sleep disturbances can, in turn, can lead to counter-productive cycles of sleeping pill administration, for both healthcare workers and patients. While in the short term it may seem like a useful quick fix, the long-term implications can be significant. For us, there can be longer-acting hangovers from some types of sedatives, impairing aspects such as judgement, concentration, and reflexes into the next day. Issues of dependence can arise quickly, be it physical or psychological. Tolerance can also develop with some medications, with, by definition, larger does required to gain the same sleep-inducing effects. And for patients, there may be an increased risk of polypharmacy interactions, and events such as falls, leading to significant complications in their recovery. If we do feel the need to prescribe a sleeping tablet, as with any medications, there needs to be careful consideration around which to prescribe, and for how long. It may also be important to remember that a sleeping tablet is not a solution in and of itself, and is more for addressing a symptom of sleeplessness in the short term. Educating patients around the need for adequate sleep, and sleep hygiene measures, may be useful. This may also help to decrease requests for sleeping tablets.

The hospital environment as a whole is generally not conducive to encouraging sleep in the patients, either. This is ironic given the restorative and recuperative roles of sleep, and its arguably having a key role in patient recovery. We should consider this, and make small changes where we can.

Chapter 3

Factor to consider: Diet

Without a doubt, many resources are stretched within healthcare systems. However, given the importance of nutrition in recovery from illness, is it important to ensure that experts such as dietitians are involved in the care of patients who require them as early as possible. It is widely recognised that good nutrition is needed for good wound healing.[13] Within this, we need adequate glucose for energy.[13] Fatty acids are needed for inflammatory processes and cell structure.[13] Decreases in collagen formation, as well as wound dehiscence and otherwise poor wound healing rates, have been associated with inadequate protein intake.[13] Similarly, vitamins are also critical for healing.

Having a low threshold in requesting the input of dietitians may be helpful. While dietitians are often in demand, and we do not wish to unnecessarily add to workloads for our colleagues, the importance of adequate nutrition cannot be overstated. Encouraging family and friends to bring in fresh fruits may also help and be appropriate in some situations, as may dietary support through prescribing supplements. Encouraging access to suitable resources such as those from the NHS online may also help the patient with education around healthy eating.

Adequate nutrition plays a key role in maintaining health, as well as in healing and recovery.

Again, without adding unnecessarily to colleagues' workloads, inpatient admissions may be a useful time for patients with chronic conditions, such as diabetes, to be seen by specialist nurses for support or a recap on aspects of managing their condition.

Factor to consider: Cognitive aspects

Thought patterns have the potential to help us or hinder us. While it is widely acknowledged that there is generally inadequate access to resources for psychological support, online resources may be helpful for some patients.

Particularly with regard conditions such as chronic pain and diabetes, online education programmes with elements around mental health may improve patient wellbeing and outcomes. Simple tools such as journaling may also be of benefit, enabling patients to reflect and also to measure their progress.

Encouraging patients to become well-informed and supported from an educational point of view about their condition may be helpful. Furthermore, we are aware of the difficulties of chronic disease, as well as the impacts of isolation, on mental health and wellbeing. Encouraging the use of specific online patient support groups or forums may be of assistance, too. So too may mindfulness techniques, as we will cover later. Discussing other tools such as the importance of goal setting, as well as referral to specialist psychological support, may also be beneficial.

Psychological support may be of benefit for patients and carers who are managing chronic conditions.

Chapter 4 **Protective factors for organisational implementation**

We need to take a multi-pronged approach in order to improve the culture of mental health awareness, action, and wellbeing for clinicians. Change can be difficult, irrespective of what level it is at. Individual behavioural change is challenging, as is change on systemic, organisational, and infrastructural levels. Yet to keep doing what we have always done, and to expect different results, is akin to insanity – according to Einstein. So, while changes may be difficult, we owe it to our patients, colleagues, and ourselves to implement small positive changes which, over time, will bring larger positive results. To cause the greatest improvements, both 'top down' as well as a 'bottom up' approaches should be used.

In order to more fully promote and protect our mental health and wellbeing, we need multi-pronged change within the healthcare systems that we work in. Organisations need to be able to make changes to promote aspects such as resilience, as well as encouraging and enabling individuals to be able to make changes, too. Changes of an organisational nature may be slowest to be implemented. Some changes merely start with a shift in attitude, which can occur as fast, or as slow, as we wish it to.

The benefits of physician-focused intervention programmes to decrease burnout may be increased by the inclusion of approaches that are directed at the organisation.[1]

In the UK, the COVID-19 pandemic highlighted just how flexible the NHS can be, with its ability to respond to the changed circumstances. In just a matter of days, hospitals were built, wards reconfigured, and rotas amended. Structural and functional change happened in a very short space of time. While this was an emergency scenario which dictated this, it did reinforce the fact that the system can be responsive. Increasing cases of healthcare practitioner burnout may also be seen as a crisis. While the changes in the NHS will likely revert to closer to what they were before, it may be an opportunity to

How to Promote Wellbeing: Practical Steps for Healthcare Practitioners' Mental Health,
First Edition. Dr Rachel K Thomas.
© 2021 Dr Rachel K. Thomas Published 2021 by John Wiley & Sons Ltd.

keep some of the current beneficial changes as a new 'set point'. It may also be helpful to keep a flexible perspective on the system, and its ability to respond to support in a particular direction as required.

Protective factor: Organisational resilience

Resilience in a healthcare setting may be complex both to conceptualise and to implement; however, that doesn't mean that we shouldn't try. We, the healthcare practitioners working within the system, may be viewed as needing to have 'individual resilience', as we will cover in Chapter 5. At present, it may be argued that there tends to be more of an emphasis on individual resilience, rather than looking to how the organisation can flex and change appropriately. However, from a systemic or organisational point of view, where the infrastructure that we work within is concerned, there is also an 'organisational resilience'. It is the ability for a system to adapt, and to flexibly respond when placed under unexpected or novel demands.

A range of processes assisted the increased resilience of the NHS during the COVID-19 crisis – its resources were augmented, as was its capacity, through recruiting staff from retirement and elective surgery pools, as well as beds from private hospitals. Convention centres were rapidly transformed into specialist centres and staff re-allocated from other areas. Yet the acute demands of a crisis, and the ongoing stretching of a healthcare system are arguably different stories. However, the rapid response has been a justified morale-booster, comfort, and source of pride for many. As mentioned, the pivoting of the system to include a range of initiatives to protect the mental health and wellbeing of those working within the system could be maintained as a new set point.

In this idea of organisational resilience, there is more of a focus on how success can be obtained and failure avoided. It looks at how we, as the healthcare practitioners working within the system, adapt and learn to create safe environments, despite the often-conflicting goals, trade-offs, and safety hazards.[2]

Looking at resilience in this way, it has several levels that are interconnected. These levels include:

- The 'individual level'. This is a more knowledge-based level, and includes individuals having the capacity to speak up and report fears about patient safety
- The 'micro-organisational level'. This is a team level, and includes clear avenues for feedback, supervised practice, and leadership
- The 'macro-organisational level'. This is the whole organisation level, and includes commitment on the corporate level to patient safety and good clinical outcomes.[3]

Chapter 4

This is a more dynamic view of resilience, and one that depends less upon its static components in the system and more upon the dynamic relationships within the system.[4] In essence it is more about what the system does and can do than about what it has in it. It has a focus that is based on how work is actually performed on the ground, rather than how it is imagined to be performed by administrators, managers, or the developers of guidelines. It has more of a focus on swift detection and anticipation of negative changes, adequate repair time if these changes do occur, or steps that can be taken to decrease the impact of such changes to minimise the amount of damage that they may cause.

Organisational resilience is a more dynamic view of resilience – more focused on the dynamic relationships than the static components.

There are three key areas of organisational resilience:

- Foresight
- Coping
- Recovery.[3]

In this context, 'foresight' is being able to see in advance that chance of something negative happening. 'Coping' relates to being able to prevent this negative occurrence from having even greater impacts or becoming worse, and 'recovery' relates to being able to recover from the negative event that has happened.

A study on clinical handovers by Jeffcott, as outlined below, puts each of these areas into context.[3] It looks at the clinical situation where there is a scheduled handover meeting between the night team and the incoming day team – and the junior doctor does not arrive. As a result, the other clinicians have to work longer to ensure continuity of care until a replacement arrives.

Breaking this down into these key areas:

Foresight (predicting something negative is happening) may occur at the time the doctor does not arrive, and steps may include:

- The individual level: contacting a replacement doctor
- The micro-organisational level: clinical supervisor identifying staffing level deficits and alerting management
- The macro-organisational level: training around handover, allocating a specific location and time for handovers.

Coping (preventing the negative event having worse impacts) may occur later, such as at the start of the next night shift, and steps may include:

- The individual level: a clinician working until a replacement arrives
- The micro-organisational level: providing a second on-call clinician as a protocol
- The macro-organisational level: day team thoroughly documenting clinical care of patients from situations of high risk overnight.

Recovery (recovering from the negative event after it has happened) may occur later still, such as at the conclusion of this next night shift, and may include:

- The individual level: clinician ensures that appropriate staff, such as supervisors, are aware of what has happened, and if there are concerns around patient care.
- The micro-organisational level: review of patients that were seen overnight; arrange cover for that clinician so as to decrease their workload.
- The macro-organisational level: review of clinical practice and of the team's management.

A framework can be used to help consider these different aspects - foresight, coping and recovery, through the individual, micro-organisational and macro-organisational lenses - in other instances (see Figure 4.1).

Research reveals that clinical handovers are often informal, prone to errors, and unstructured, and that the majority of doctors see benefit in making this process more formalised.[5]

Other high-risk industries look more to how teams and organisations act in situations where a breakdown or failure occurs in their high-risk

	foresight	coping	recovery
individual			
micro			
macro			

Figure 4.1 A framework for considering key areas of organisation resilience.[3]

situations. As part of this, they may have a more formal or structured analysis of issues that occur and may focus on 'Why did things go *right*?' rather than 'Why did things go *wrong*?'. This may lead to concentrating on proactively recovering from errors, rather than simply reacting to errors that have been made.[3]

The evidence supports that micro- and macro-organisational-level interventions may help with clinicians' mental health aspects in healthcare practitioners, too. A recent meta-analysis looked at the evidence around interventions to help reduce burnout, specifically in physicians.[1] This found that interventions aimed at the organisational level, or directed by the organisation, showed effects that were improved significantly as compared to interventions that were directed by the physicians, or aimed at the physician level, alone. It concluded that programmes aiming to deliver interventions for physicians to decrease burnout were associated with benefits that were small, yet these may be boosted with the use of approaches that were directed at the organisational level. It also concluded the idea that 'burnout is a problem of the whole health care organisation, rather than individuals'.[1]

Many current interventions for mental health and wellbeing focus on the individual clinician. The responsibility is placed on us, with relatively little comment as to how our healthcare organisations can be improved.[6] However, improved support and a more optimal system to work within would go a long way in preventing the triggering of these stresses in the first place. Improved support systems after an event may go a long way towards decreasing longer term and second wave impacts.

An organisation's 'safety culture' and its 'mindfulness' are factors required to be integrated for an organisation to be resilient in this way.[3]

'Safety culture' is often discussed in healthcare organisations. It relates to 'safe' work being the priority, as in the safety of the overall work environment. The different levels – the individual, the micro-organisational, and the macro-organisational – all prioritise this. This priority is evident in the daily occurrences of the healthcare organisation, through the attitudes and actions of those involved in it. For example, there is a clear need to look at how shortages in the workforce increase the impact of already growing workloads, which adds to the stresses for clinicians in the first place.[6] Or the lack of adequate PPE leading to reluctance to go to work for fear of inadequate protection from communicable diseases, as highlighted in the recent pandemic.

By comparison, 'mindfulness' looks at individuals in an organisation having a greater awareness of what is occurring in the environment around them. It is commonly discussed in relation to an individual, as we will cover later, and there is a significant body of evidence supporting its benefits.

However, the idea of this concept being applied to organisations such as a healthcare system is newer and less researched. In this definition, there is a greater vigilance around noticing risk, and this is at the forefront of individuals' minds. It involves constantly monitoring safety aspects, with the intention of noticing anything 'out of the ordinary' as quickly as possible and stopping developments in an unhelpful direction – hopefully before a negative significant event occurs as an action trigger. Given preconceptions attached to the word 'mindfulness', 'sensitive surveillance' may be a more suitable name.

Therefore, it may be suggested that promoting resilience is a multifactorial issue in healthcare – that it is not only the problem of the individuals, us, the practitioners working within the system, but also the problem of the system that we, individuals, are working within, too.

Protective factor: Organisational approaches to addressing stigmatisation

As already mentioned, stigma is a complex and multi-dimensional process. There is no one-size-fits-all solution for it – perhaps ironic, given that this kind of generic 'one-size-fits-all' response often stems from stereotyped views.

There are various levels within healthcare systems that can be affected by stigmatisation – the structural, the interpersonal, and even the intraindividual.[7] This also means that there are multiple areas for potential improvement. For instance, structural levels may relate to how resources are invested and organisational culture. Interpersonal may include negative and discriminatory behaviours, while intraindividual may relate to feeling reluctant to seek support or disclose a pre-existing mental health diagnosis.[7]

Research shows that the reduction of stigma in healthcare settings needs to be approached with a clear goal of changing culture, with an approach that is both integrated and sustained and tackles both inward-facing and out-ward facing aspects.[7] Using participation that is incentivised, or even mandatory, as well as using measures related to stigma-reduction in the quality of care metrics have also been emphasised.[7] Skills-based education programmes, teaching person-first behaviours, through lessons on 'what to do and say', may also help. This is recognised as a different kind of interaction which we may have with our patients, or socially with colleagues.

Having mental health and wellbeing strategies embedded into aspects such as line management may also help.[8] This approach of standardising these aspects, so that they are a common aspect in training, may help to address stigma. Ensuring that managers and administration staff are well trained in how to have conversations that relate to mental health may help. This may be as simple as an online course and a practical component to enable these skills to be practised. Furthermore, also ensuring that these staff members are aware of how to refer colleagues for additional support, as well as being trained to provide some basic guidance around workplace wellbeing, may help, too.[8]

Similarly, workplaces should have a zero-tolerance attitude to bullying. The previously highly hierarchical nature of healthcare and medicine has shifted, from paternalistic to patient-centric, and attitudes within the system need to evolve, too. This involves creating systems and policies to enable an 'equal voice' within teams, such that any team member feels that they can voice their thoughts and opinions without concerns of being victimised or overlooked. It may also involve facilitating the safe reporting of issues, without fear of repercussions on the reporter, as discussed in whistleblowing.

Protective factor: Creating a culture of support[9]

Clarifying and then promoting shared values in the workforce may help support mental health and wellbeing. Being clear on our common goal and values helps align our actions towards achieving these. Ensuring that we take steps to encourage a sense of enjoyment at work, and helping ourselves and our colleagues to feel fulfilled in the work that they do each day may help.

Enabling clinicians to have the flexibility to amend work hours at certain times may also help. While this may mean that staff rotas and rosters need additional staff or allocation changes to balance this, given the potential to improve patient care as well as the wellbeing of the workforce, this may be a comparably small administrative and financial cost to pay.

Empowering the workforce to be involved in the initiatives in the workplace that are promoting and protecting their mental health and wellbeing may also be of benefit. This may be as simple as enabling initiatives to be suggested in a streamlined manner, through to facilitating trials of staff-led ideas. Promoting clinicians who are on the 'front line' to suggest what may work for them may understandably lead to different suggestions to those from colleagues in a more managerial role. Furthermore, promoting involvement in the design of mental health and wellbeing policy design may increase the likelihood of support and participation in such initiatives.

Encouraging a workplace that is free from blame allocation may also be a valuable component of creating a supportive workplace culture. While it is inevitable that errors and poor outcomes may occur, being able to learn from these in a way that is not associated with blame allocation is key – not only for improving the mental health of those involved, but also for encouraging open dialogue around systems to help protect against similar instances occurring again.

Taking choices that lead to a range of smaller changes can help to create a culture of greater support.

Effort to ensure that the workplace pressures, as well as the risks associated with some workplace areas, are kept to a minimum is also key. These can help to combine together to help minimise sources of ill-health for those working there.

Encouraging more conversations around mental health issues at work may also help. It may help to normalise how these are perceived. Speaking about our feelings of stress may also help our colleagues who may have difficulty, for various reasons, in speaking about this. As previously mentioned, there is still a large stigma around clinicians admitting that they have a mental health diagnosis, as well as delays and reluctance around seeking help for mental health signs. Creating clearer, smoother paths to enable clinicians to access help – be it anonymously or otherwise – may help. Greater signposting around how to quickly and efficiently access support in times of need may also be of benefit. Aiming to normalise behaviours associated with seeking help for mental health concerns, as well as encouraging those who are concerned, may be of benefit. Furthermore, active attempts to raise awareness of our own mental health as well as those around us may help to create a more supportive culture. This may include training courses or other education, as well as colleagues who are mental health 'leads'.

Research shows that junior doctors are the most likely to state they haven't been made aware of the appropriate ways to access support.[9] In this same research, almost 10% of the respondents stated they had not been offered support by their medical school or employer despite asking for it (Figure 4.2).[9] Almost 20% of respondents stated they would not ask for support at their place of work, training, or study (Figure 4.3).

Working in hospitals can mean that at times we are involved in, or bear witness to, traumatic events. These may range from violent injuries and deaths in patients to transitions in our career. Creating an environment where we feel supported at these times, as well as improving our ability to recognise these times, may be helpful.

'Wobble rooms', rooms to where any healthcare practitioners could retreat privately if they were feeling particularly emotional, were introduced during the recent pandemic. Many hospitals already provide designated offices for healthcare teams to meet and chat; however, the additional wobble rooms

Chapter 4

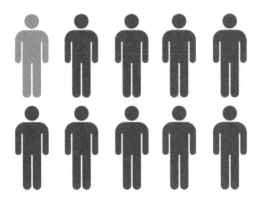

Figure 4.2 Almost 10% (9%) of the respondents stated that they had not been offered support by their medical school or employer despite asking for it just the number.[9]

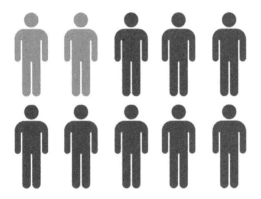

Figure 4.3 Almost 20% (19%) of respondents stated that they would not ask for support at their place of work, training, or study.[9]

were intended to facilitate a moment away even from colleagues if needed – with the idea that 'it's okay to have a wobble'. They also provided staff with a location for access to resources, such as support hotlines.

Feeling supported enough to have conversations on mental health and wellbeing, and access to services with educational supervisors, is of particular benefit to junior clinicians, who are at higher risk of burnout. Additionally, encouraging colleagues, and having a low threshold for seeking out support after stressful incidents, should be encouraged. This may also involve encouraging routine reflection on stressful events, as will be discussed later.

The BMA released a Mental Wellbeing Charter in response to reports on the high levels of burnout in clinicians having been published.[10] This Charter called for healthcare employers to take steps such as:

- 'Embed staff wellbeing into the organisational culture
- Tackle the mental health stigma and encourage staff to seek help if needed
- Provide access to high-quality support services
- Better support managers in identifying signs and symptoms of poor mental health in staff
- Encourage staff to take breaks
- Provide spaces for staff to rest and socialise.'[10]

Their recommendations also included the idea that a 'Wellbeing Guardian' be appointed at NHS board-level roles, responsible for focusing on the wellbeing of staff members, and that active means of commuting to work be encouraged by the inclusion of showers in hospital facilities. Similarly, simple steps can be taken to try to promote other aspects of wellbeing, such as the ability to have meal breaks. While obviously patient emergencies cannot be predicted, and these are the priority, may other aspects of healthcare jobs – even in hospitals – can be prioritised. For instance, all healthcare teams can be made aware of trying to protect each other's break time, such as not bleeping for routine or non-urgent tasks during this time. Many hospitals have protected teaching time for students and trainees – and offering food at these can help to both ensure a meal is eaten, and that the session is attended!

Part of this culture of support should include support not only at work, but also on the return to work after illness or absence. The BMA Charter also recommends programmes to encourage mentoring or coaching.[8] A buddying system for junior doctors may be helpful in increasing feelings of connection.[8] It is important for there to be clear leadership for the wellbeing initiatives. Staff need to 'lead by example', as well as creating environments where both staff and students feel valued.[8] Offering training on how to effectively communicate, as well as how to debrief effectively, may help.

Protective factor: Facilitating access and awareness of support avenues

Many healthcare systems already provide some types of support mechanisms for staff. There is usually room for improvement, however, and the first step is to identify and access what is already available.

Conversations on mental health and how to access support should start early in our careers. It is important that in early training, such as at medical school, a more proactive attitude is encouraged. This may include conversations reassuring students that if they do seek help through support services, it will not lead to adverse effects on their career.

Occupational health services may be able to offer some support, or provide directions to existing resources in the particular hospital where we are working. Adequate promotion, such as posters, intranet bulletins, or emails, of what is available is also useful. Clearly signposting how to access this support may well decrease any barriers to actually accessing it.

We are so used to working under stress, assuming this is a 'part of the job', that guidelines on when to seek help, along with other awareness raising suggestions, may be useful. Encouraging colleagues to use the available services, in a supportive manner, may help, as may the appointment of a specifically trained mental health first-aider.

The types of support services that are created for clinicians may need to be amended from other more traditional services or those that are already in place. Given the nature of our workflow, the support may need to be accessed at different times, may need to be able to be accessed quickly, and given the stigma that some may feel is associated with accessing services, may need to be able to be accessed confidentially. Given the rates of addiction amongst clinicians, access to services designed for this may be of benefit.

Simple practical lifestyle measures, such as ensuring separate space for clinicians to have a break and prepare food or tea, are important. Allocating a break space for sustenance, as well as conversations away from patients, may help to encourage reflections on clinical instances, as well as other topics. While many hospitals do have this, it is important to recognise their value and to therefore preserve them.

Protective factor: Promoting communication

It goes almost without saying that communication is critical for clinicians. Effective communication with staff who may have been on leave, with an agreed frequency, and steps to promote their return to work is also key. So too is induction for new staff, which many hospitals now have as standard policy. Review meetings for how staff are progressing with returning to work after a period of absence may also be of benefit.[8] While meetings and discussions take time in already time-pressured days, it may also be beneficial to recognise these as opportunities for key learning and CPD for all parties involved.

Furthermore, good quality clinical care for patients is closely linked to communication. Between teams such as primary and specialist care, communication that is written is the most prevalent form.[11] Inpatient interactions are commonly face-to-face, while with other teams in hospital they may vary to include over the telephone, as in response to bleeps. The importance of aspects such as nonverbal communication is referred to in Chapter 6.

Promoting conversations after critical or concerning incidents between staff members may also be of benefit, as is covered more fully in Chapter 7. It may not only help those affected in understanding and managing their feelings and stresses; it may also provide a learning opportunity to prevent it happening again. After crises such as the COVID-19 pandemic, ensuring that there are safe, inclusive, and confidential frameworks for debriefing, as well as ensuring that there is the time and capacity to do so, is important.

Different types of communication groups may be of benefit in reflective discussions. The BMA Charter recommended access to talking groups such as:

- Schwartz rounds
- Balint groups.[8]

A Schwartz round is a type of reflective practice that is in a group forum. It enables reflection on emotional aspects.[12] Evaluation of these rounds reported that staff found they had value in enabling mental processing of challenges in the workplace, as well as decreasing their feelings of isolation.[13] It also found that regular attendance halved the proportion of participants with psychological wellbeing that was poor, according to the General Health Questionnaire (GHQ 12).[14]

A Balint group is a small group of participants (6–12) meeting to confidentially and non-judgementally discuss patient interactions for approximately one hour.[15] A trained leader helps guide the group, specifically focusing on how the interactions have made the healthcare practitioner feel, with the goal being to help increase understanding around this as well as patient–doctor relationships.[15] These groups may help enable reflection and support, with reports of increased job satisfaction due to the groups potentially helping to decrease burnout.

Protective factor: Balancing the psychosocial safety climate

Considering the psychosocial safety climate (PSC) that we work within may have a large impact on how we handle workplace stress and is also therefore linked to burnout. The PSC relates to the workplace climate for safety and psychological health, and inherently reflects how productivity weighs against management's concerns about psychological health.[16] The levels of psychosocial risk factors are high in health services sectors, as are the psychological health problems in this area.[16] The PSC relates to risks that are linked to management, as well as the type of work that we do, including factors such as its social context.[17] While the PSC may be linked closely to how much

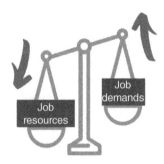

Figure 4.4   Our stress at work can be linked to the balance between the resources available and the demands present.

work stress we experience, it may also help to highlight ways that we may improve this – both on an individual as well as an organisational level.

> 'Psychosocial safety climate (PSC) is defined as shared perceptions of organisational policies, practices, and procedures for the protection of worker psychological health and safety that stem largely from management practices.'[18]

Evidence supports that developing a PSC that is robust may help to buffer against the effects of psychosocial hazards in workplaces, including that it may moderate against job demands' effects on depression.[19]

How we cope with the demands of our job as clinicians is affected by aspects of PSC (Figure 4.4). One model defines work life in six areas.[20]

- Workload
- Reward
- Control
- Values
- Fairness
- Community.

One aspect is the workload itself – the nature of the work, the quantity, and the demands that this places on us. However, aspects which contribute to the PSC include not only the workload that is experienced, but also how much control we feel we have over this workload – and our workday.

Similarly, the sense of reward that we obtain, the amount of job satisfaction that we glean, can impact on the PSC. The presence of a sense of community, and how connected we feel to this, may also have an impact. The fairness and values that are displayed within the organisation also have an impact on the PSC – if we feel subject to discrimination, this can count against it.

There are aspects that can therefore be addressed within each of these areas, so that the conditions can be made more favourable. Feelings that a workload is disproportionate to capabilities or time may be a risk; however, there may be some flexibility with adjusting workloads through processes such as effective delegation or teamwork. A workplace that seems unfair due to the impression of favouritism or discrimination would obviously benefit if these were to be addressed through processes and policy changes.

The sense of control that is felt around aspects such as hours and the sense of autonomy around decisions in the workday may vary – we cannot predict when an emergency will come through the door, or a previously stable patient will deteriorate. However, having backups or processes in place to support this, or having other days where we are able to have more control, may help to balance this.

A sense of community, for instance working within a team, may also help. As mentioned, the idea of buddying or mentoring programmes may help, particularly in new or particularly high-stress environments. And this sense of community may be fostered through reflective practices, as will be discussed, or informally through chatting over a cup of tea. Reflecting on a 'common mission' may also help with feeling part of being on the same team, even if working in more isolation.

Healthcare systems should aim to regularly promote support services and ensure that clear guidance is offered on how to access these – particularly emphasising that these services can be accessed confidentially.[8] It is also key that they ensure that these services can be accessed in a manner that accommodates the working hours and shift patterns of those that need them.[8] And there also should be an effective method for evaluating how the services are used, and how effectively they are meeting the expectations and requirements of those that are using them.[8]

Recommendations around the provision of services, according to the BMA Charter is that these services be either in house or external, with self-referral options, offering:

- Psychological counselling
- Addiction counselling
- Occupational health services that are confidential and comprehensive.[8]

Where possible, staff input on the layout of working areas and common areas should be sought. This may help to decrease the risk of workplace harm.[8] Where possible, areas should be designed to enable staff to take a break outdoors, too.[8] According to this BMA Charter, other key areas in helping to provide a healthy, safe workplace may include:

- Ensuring that there is access to drinking water
- Ensuring that there is nutritious food available
- Providing access to car-parking, particularly for staff who work shifts at night
- Ensuring that there is access to break rooms for communication, food preparation, and rest
- Promoting activities such as an active commute to work, and providing showers and lockers to facilitate this.[8]

And even apparently simple strategies, such as including a drinking fountain near a clinicians' common area may help – as seeing the fountain acts as a visual reminder, promoting adequate hydration.

Protective factor: Implementing a wellbeing strategy

As discussed, appointing staff members who have a focus on promoting and protecting staff wellbeing – for example as a 'Wellbeing Guardian' – may be a helpful step in implementing a wellbeing strategy.

Included within such a strategy could be recognising and linking to the objectives of the healthcare organisation, providing a plan for implementation, providing clear engagement metrics and resources and support from management levels.[8] Developing methods and processes for monitoring and reporting back to management on the impact of such interventions would also be useful.[8] As such, the wellbeing interventions would need to be measured against pre-determined objectives, with feedback being included to enable the efficacy of these interventions to be understood, and to suggest how to iterate them for greater impact.

There may need to be recognition of a broad number of ways to engage with different members of the workforce who may have different needs – there is no 'one-size-fits-all' strategy, as discussed. But by having staff who are specifically focused on implementing effective strategies, there may be an improvement in impact.

Part of implementing a wellbeing strategy may mean that general steps in creating a culture that is supportive of wellbeing and staff mental health may need to be taken. Broader aspects, as covered elsewhere in this book in more depth but highlighted in the BMA Charter include:

- Preventing and treating causes of poorer wellbeing
- Promoting discussions around mental health and the available support options
- Planning, producing, and putting in place effective policies.[8]

Aspects of preventing and remedying causes of that are detrimental to wellbeing may include aiming to evaluate the risks that staff are currently under and how to manage these, as well as encouraging staff to take breaks, eat and drink during shifts, and to engage in healthy lifestyle behaviours. It highlights that acute care should not be scheduled at a time that conflicts with lunch where possible, and that 'regular wellbeing check-ins' could be useful.[8] In order to help promote conversations around mental health and wellbeing, steps should be taken to both encourage and normalise behaviours related to seeking help, as well as help create safe environments for discussion around mental health.[8] While complicated to implement, encouragement of flexible working options, as well as an active focus on promoting more balance between work and life, may also help with building this culture.

Having training around the importance of recovery behaviours, and having breaks included in timetables and frameworks, may also help. Aiming to create work environments where breaks are regarded as the norm will be a process; however, anecdotal evidence supports that in the interim, many healthcare practitioners would cover a colleague's workload so that they can take a break.

And, as a part of putting effective policies in place, these need to be reviewed and adapted as required to ensure that they are meeting the required goals and expectations. Many other areas have key performance indicators (KPI), and using a KPI system for wellbeing could also be of benefit.

Chapter 4

Chapter 5 **Protective factors for individual implementation**

Many factors, including our lifestyles, affect our individual mental health and wellbeing. We may have more control over these factors, and a greater ability to improve them more rapidly, than we have with controlling organisational factors. Nevertheless, some aspects of our lifestyle may be hard to change. We need to be aware that promoting and protecting mental health and wellbeing lies not only as a responsibility of each individual, but also with the organisation. As we champion the use of multi-disciplinary teams (MDTs) for the most effective care of our patients, so too may a multi-dimensional approach be the most effective for us, too.

Protective factor: Learning a new wellbeing skill

Learning to manage our own wellbeing can be thought of as an important skill – one that can help improve our own lifestyle, health, and career, as well as improve outcomes for the patients we are caring for. When we are considering our own wellbeing behaviours, it can be helpful to review theory on the stages of learning, which breaks down how we learn new skills, and provides a framework applicable to any new skill. Not all of us will regard learning these new behaviours as skills, or reflect on them in this way, but we can gain insight into what we are doing and how we can improve things for ourselves by becoming more aware of where we currently stand on this scale (Figure 5.1).

Stage one is *unconscious incompetence*. This is basically where we have no idea about how to do something new but have no idea that we have no idea – 'blissful ignorance'. At this stage, we are unaware that we need to do something differently, or how it could be done. This ignorance is holding us back from consciously developing a new and useful skill.

Stage two is *conscious incompetence*. Here we understand that we don't have the required skills to do something. This stage is difficult for some of us,

How to Promote Wellbeing: Practical Steps for Healthcare Practitioners' Mental Health,
First Edition. Dr Rachel K. Thomas.
© 2021 Dr Rachel K. Thomas. Published 2021 by John Wiley & Sons Ltd.

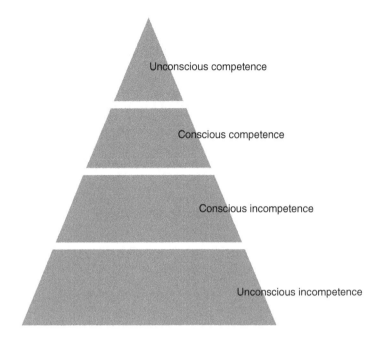

Figure 5.1 The stages of competence when learning a new skill.

particularly those who have an overly perfectionistic attitude to themselves or their work, a not uncommon trait with clinicians. During this stage we may even judge ourselves harshly or negatively for not being able to perform the skills we have in mind. This stage often precedes a more dedicated effort to learn something. However, given that this extra effort will be required, people may give up on learning the new skill at this stage.

Stage three is *conscious competence*. This relates to knowing that we know how to do something. This can also be an effortful or uncomfortable stage for many of us.

And the final stage of learning is stage four, *unconscious competence*. This is where the skill we have been learning is basically 'second nature'. We do not have to think about doing it. It may feel like an ingrained behaviour, and does not have the self-consciousness related to it that the previous two stages of learning may have. It is at this stage when our newly learned skill becomes easier, and more automatic, for us.

Reflecting on our position in this framework in relation to skills and processes for promoting and protecting our mental health and wellbeing is useful for several reasons. Firstly, it helps us have a more goal-focused and achievement-based view of what we are trying to learn. Secondly, it helps provide motivation – if we are finding it difficult to learn a new skill, identifying that we are at a recognisably 'difficult' stage helps us by knowing that others find it difficult at this stage too, and that later stages will require less effort.

Protective factor: Defining motivation to change

The recognised high rates of burnout, with consequent negative impact on patient care and outcomes, provides a logical reason for developing skills that promote and protect our wellbeing. However, what actually motivates each of us to put in the effort to change is highly personal and multi-factorial.

Being clear on the reasons for changing behaviour may help to maintain new behaviours when times are challenging.

Common reasons for people to start thinking about need for change, and steps to take, include:

- A critical life event, such as an illness or change in circumstance such as getting fired
- Levels of distress – for example, a severe period of anxiety may prompt change
- Recognition of the negative consequences of continuing in the same manner
- External incentives that may be either positive and/or negative
- Cognitive appraisal or evaluation, such as weighing up the 'pros and cons' of continuing certain behaviours.[1]

Spending a moment to reflect on where we are, and what our motivations to change are, will encourage us to instigate, and then hopefully maintain, the necessary behaviours for change. Has there been a critical incident that we were involved in? Are we receiving negative feedback from our personal relationships on any of our work, or home, behaviours? Are we feeling too tired to engage in activities that we usually enjoy? Clarifying *why* we want to change aspects of how we are currently managing our mental health and wellbeing may help us with the motivation to define, carry out, and then act consistently on, steps to help us.

A structured and evidence-based method of behavioural change is through *motivational interviews*. This is a way of trying to understand the mechanisms behind behavioural change.[2] A primary principle of a motivational interview is that the person desiring or requiring the changes raises the reasons for a change in behaviour, not the counsellor or therapist. Such techniques may be used by mental health professionals, but an in-depth analysis of them is beyond the scope of this book. However, it is useful for us to reflect on what we would like to change, what happens if we do not change, and what happens if we do.

Behaviour I'd like to change	What happens if I don't change	What happens with change

Having a clear idea of *why* we want to put in the effort to make changes in our lifestyle or to improve our wellbeing can help, particularly when we are feeling that it is just 'all too hard' to make the change. While a motivation for change may not be useful in affecting external factors which are influencing us, it may well help with how we respond to those factors, and how we interact with those factors which we are able to change.

Protective factor: Individual resilience

Resilience is our ability to be able to cope with, and adapt to, stress and adversity successfully.[3] It includes how we are able to basically 'bounce back' despite things not going our way.

Resilience = successfully adapting through adversity and stress

It relates to how we can maintain a 'normal' degree of physical and mental functioning even when faced with stresses, adversity, and things basically not going as planned, or 'not going our way'.

Post-traumatic stress disorder (PTSD), depression, and other mental health conditions can develop from chronic adversity and trauma, as we have previously discussed. These conditions do not develop in some individuals, even when they have been subjected to the same trauma, as explained by the diathesis-stress model. Developing effective coping strategies and responses for negatively changing environments may help buffer and moderate our responses to these stresses. While this may not necessarily fully protect us from mental health conditions or negative outcomes developing in association with the stress that we have been exposed to, in some of us, it may help.

Evidence shows that many factors are involved in the development of resilience. Some factors that can enhance resilience include:

- Social factors
- Psychological factors
- Developmental factors
- Genetic factors
- Epigenetic factors
- Biological factors.

A recent meta-analysis on resilience and its relationship to aspects in personality showed that neuroticism and resilience were negatively correlated.[4]

A study looking at the resilience of workers in the NHS found higher levels of resilience in older employees and in those who were working 18–38 hours per week, and lower levels in clinical staff. Interestingly this study found no correlation between resilience levels and rates of absence.[5] Another study, comparing high stress jobs and absence rates, also found a lack of correlation between the two, but, however, concluded that short absences may actually be used by 'hardy' individuals as a 'positive coping strategy'.[6] This indicates that both presenteeism and absenteeism may actually be negative coping strategies.

Protecting factor: Compassion satisfaction and self-care

Being compassionate in how we deliver clinical care is linked to better outcomes for our patients.[7] A meta-analysis of 11 studies (approximately 4,000 participants) showed interesting associations with compassion satisfaction, the rewards that we feel when we are helping to care for others. This research found a strong correlation between burnout and compassion fatigue. Compassion satisfaction was shown to be weakly associated in a protective way against compassion fatigue, and moderately protective against burnout. Compassion satisfaction also had a moderately positive association with a positive affect (an 'immediate expression of emotion') and slightly decreased burnout.[8] Interestingly, compassion satisfaction was not significantly correlated to professional factors, demographic factors, burnout, or compassion fatigue.

So, if the evidence shows that compassion satisfaction moderately decreases burnout, how can we promote compassion satisfaction? There is significantly more research into compassion fatigue than specifically into compassion satisfaction. With compassion fatigue, research indicates that it commonly has four themes.[7]

- The trigger –an *'unbearable weight on shoulders'*
- The prevention – *'who has my back?'*
- The emotional – *'walking on a tightrope'*
- The physical – *'just plain worn out'*.[9]

In order to promote compassion satisfaction, we could well start by addressing these points.

A small study (n=37) of doctors working in hospice settings, undoubtedly high-stress environments, explored the relationship between compassion satisfaction and self-care.[10] It found that those doctors with strategies for self-care displayed greater compassion satisfaction, as well as having lesser compassion fatigue and burnout. The self-care strategies included:

- Workplace
- Physical
- Emotional
- Psychological
- Spiritual
- Balance.[10]

Self-care practices by these doctors included speaking with co-workers, regular eating, permitting time to cry, ensuring reflection, finding inspiring aspects, and aiming for balance in different areas such as family and work-life.[10] Self-care strategies vary, but *'as a training domain, self-care is a spectrum of knowledge, skills, and attitudes including self-reflection and self-awareness, identification and prevention of burnout, appropriate professional boundaries, and grief and bereavement'*.[11]

Some medical bodies are starting to include education or guidance on the management of sleep; however, self-care *per se* still receives relatively little direct attention. Interestingly, self-care is starting to be included as a specific competency in some areas, such as Hospice and Palliative Medicine.[11] These guidelines cover topics such as how to recognise the signs of burnout not only in ourselves but also in others, self-awareness, self-reflection, and self-care planning.[11]

The idea of self-care can be divided up into several areas, including professional and personal areas (Figure 5.2).[11] In breaking self-care into sections, we obtain more clearly-defined areas to focus on and a clearer pathway for how to do this.

Chapter 5

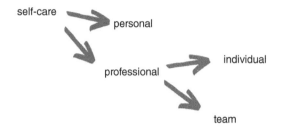

Figure 5.2 The division of self-care into groups to facilitate improvement.

Strategies for personal self-care start with the awareness that life is composed of numerous different facets beyond work. While it does include our work, it also includes the community that we are a part of, our families, how we feel internally, and our spiritual aspects. Identifying and reflecting on how we are feeling currently in these different areas of our life helps us to identify areas where we could make some change in order to improve our wellbeing. There are many different ways for us to self-care, including putting effort into the relationships that matter to us, prioritising enough sleep, exercise, and a healthy diet, taking steps supportive of our spiritual beliefs, and fostering meditative practices and mindfulness.[11]

It is helpful if we consider the various areas of our life – our physical and mental health, our work life and finances, and our social and romantic relationships. We can identify how satisfied we are in different areas of our life by using a *target* (Figure 5.3). If we feel very satisfied, we can make a mark close to the centre of the target, and if we are less satisfied, a mark for this area can be placed more peripherally. For example, Figure 5.3 shows a greater level of satisfaction in romantic relationship and physical health, than in social relationships and work life. The least satisfaction is evident in the areas of mental health and finances.

We can identify how we feel we are currently going in different areas of our own life by using the target shown in Figure 5.4. By marking where we are currently in each of the specified areas, we get an indication of what we are least satisfied with, which we can then put more effort into improving.

We commonly deliver patient care in a multi-disciplinary team (MDT), where both a team and individuals contribute to the patient's treatment. This approach is useful to apply as an analogy for our own self-care, too. With a multi-pronged approach, further divided into individual and team components, we can optimise our wellbeing.

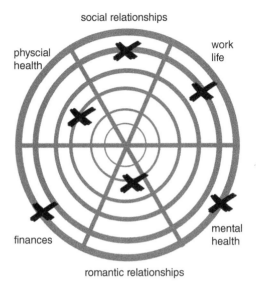

Figure 5.3   Key areas of life, and our satisfaction in them, can be represented diagrammatically.

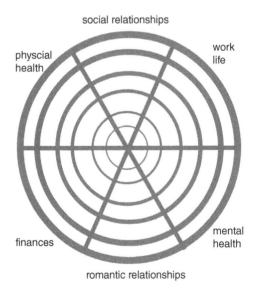

Figure 5.4   Reflecting on these key areas can indicate where we can make improvements - we can try our own reflection here.

Individual professional self-care examples include:

- Regularly considering and appraising work areas
- Creating a supportive group of mentors
- Creating a supportive group of peers
- Searching for opportunities to engage with workplace organisations
- Working on skills such as communication skills
- Focusing on self-awareness
- Creating boundaries and limits to prevent work overload
- Actively engaging in reflective practices such as writing.[11]

Team professional self-care considers how the structure and inherent processes within a work team influences its wellbeing.[11] Examples of how to improve this include:

- Initiatives to increase how we empathise with others in our team
- Guidance and protocols around team meetings
- Communicating the ways we find helpful working within our team.

Protective factor: Promoting individual action

We are well-placed to notice changes in our colleagues, given the amount of time we spend with them at work. It is helpful to be aware of the signs and symptoms of stress or mental health conditions, and of how we can instigate conversations on these, if required, with our colleagues. Effective ways to offer support if a colleague needs help may be as simple as starting a conversation.

It is important to encourage staff to be responsible for their *own* mental health and wellbeing. A key part of this is to create an environment where people feel encouraged to value their own health and wellbeing, and that any steps they take to promote and protect this will be respected rather than mocked, obstructed, or criticised. Helping workers acknowledge the avenues that are available for support, and communicating how they might access them, may also help. It is also important that there is an awareness of how difficult it may be for some of us to recognise or accept help – and how important it is to strive to be empathetic if we recognise our colleagues are in this situation.

We can all take actions towards creating an inclusive workplace, where feedback is welcomed, encouraged, and appropriately acted upon. We know that organisational change can significantly impact our mental health and wellbeing. However, our individual wise choices can cause change more rapidly, and may even lead to favourable institutional change.

Protective factor: Awareness and mitigation of risk factors for burnout

As already covered, conversations around burnout are not intended to highlight failures in or by an individual. They are intended to focus on the tipping point that any one of us may reach after periods of stress, or after a range of other factors that may be linked to burnout – including aspects of the institutions that we work in.

Workplaces where there are excessively long hours, work overload, emotionally taxing interactions, fatigue, minimal amounts of self-direction and autonomy, mentally demanding work, and changes to clinical practice from organisational levels make burnout increasingly likely.[12] Despite this sounding like a standard day at work for many of us!

There are certain areas of work environments that may lower stress levels for those working in them, and given that burnout is related to workplace stress, this may be of benefit in reducing burnout. Some of these positive work attributes include family–work balance (for example, childcare services), leadership that is competent, professional development opportunities, individual satisfaction (for example, feeling that patients appreciate what we are doing for them), and the functionality of the organisation (such as how effective and efficient the communication is).[13]

Being young, female, unmarried, and working long hours in a job that brings little satisfaction, are greater risk factors for burnout.[14] While some of these factors cannot be modified, being aware of the increased risk associated with them, or the increased risk to other colleagues, may help in having steps taken earlier in order to decrease future burnout risk. Studies support that working excessively long hours leaves individuals at higher vulnerability for emotional and psychological disturbances. Around 90% of clinicians stated that the studying, working, and training environment contributed to that their condition, with older doctors more likely to state this.[15]

The degree of interference our work has with our family life, or our work–life balance, is a potentially modifiable factor. Several studies found that this may be a contributor to burnout in doctors. One study of specialists found that work interfering with home life was one of the aspects most related to stress, along with not living up to professional standards.[16] Studies have shown that higher levels of burnout are associated with lower levels of job satisfaction.[17] However, this relationship is complex, since 'high burnout' specialties do not necessarily have the lowest levels of work–life balance or satisfaction.

There are a range of modifiable risk factors for burnout, and addressing these may help to decrease the risk of burnout.

Chapter 5

Obviously, some factors which put us at a higher risk of burnout are modifiable, while others are not. For instance, any increased risk associated with gender and age is not immediately modifiable. However, with knowledge of this increased risk, we can be more aware and open to offering, or accepting, the appropriate support. We can be more alert in looking for the signs and symptoms indicating that we, or a work colleague, is at a point where they would benefit from interventions. There is also potential to modify the impact of other risk factors. These modifications may be through behavioural change, such as increasing protective factors, and through recovery behaviours.

When resources are chronically stretched in healthcare systems, it can be left up to the clinicians to patch up the expanded requirements of the system in order to prevent it collapsing altogether. Logically, this cannot go on indefinitely. Reflecting on recruitment numbers for UK healthcare highlights the point. Senior physicians state that nearly 1,400 advertised consultant posts have led to only 800 being appointed.[18] They also estimated that 25% of doctors are lost between medical school and consultant level, and of those that do practise as a consultant, many choose early retirement due to work pressures. Some also state that with increasing numbers of admissions, yet decreasing numbers of hospital beds, the only way to keep the healthcare system functioning is with early discharges and short hospital stays. Again, logically, there must be a limit to this, and this limit is more rapidly reached in times of crisis.

Protective factor: Recognising and intervening approaching burnout and compassion fatigue

As we approach burnout, patient safety and quality of care may start to decrease. These may be warning signs that may be noticed with either subjective feedback, such as comments from colleagues, or objective feedback, such as morbidity data. Approaching burnout may be linked with an increase in the number of complaints we receive, and could be coupled with an increase in our medicolegal risk, too. Feeling lower levels of satisfaction with our work, or feeling depleted emotionally, are warning signs of possible burnout.

As already mentioned, we can use the MBI to help us identify and measure our risk of burnout. The MBI captures the three dimensions: personal accomplishment, depersonalisation, and emotional exhaustion.

The inventory is available under licence; however, a rough proxy for how we are feeling relates to how much energy we feel we have, our attitudes to work and patients, and how satisfied we are feeling with our work.

Maslach's dimension	Personal accomplishment	Depersonalisation	Emotional exhaustion
How is your. . .?	sense of satisfaction?	attitude of detachment?	energy level?
Greater burnout risk	Decreasing score	Increasing score	Increasing score

Asking ourselves these questions will help us determine our risk of burnout.
- How satisfied am I feeling with the work that am doing? Do I feel like a valued part of my team, delivering care that is worthwhile?

If we are feeling a decreasing amount of satisfaction, it could indicate a feeling of decreasing 'personal accomplishment'.
- How is my attitude to my patients? Do I catch myself thinking things like 'work would be great, were it not for the patients. . .'? Do I feel I need to try to protect myself from my patients by detaching or withdrawing, or perhaps starting to see them less as people and more as objects?

If we are feeling an increasing amount of these feelings, it may indicate an increasing sense of 'depersonalisation'.
- How do I feel at the end of the day – am I feeling emotionally drained and empty? Do I feel like people are making more demands on my emotions than I am capable of delivering?

If we are feeling an increase in these types of emotion, it may indicate an increase in our 'emotional exhaustion'. The higher the Emotional Exhaustion and Depersonalisation scores, and the lower the Personal Accomplishment score, the more we may be at risk of suffering from burnout.

There are obviously many signs and symptoms that we may notice in ourselves or in our colleagues due to burnout. A brief checklist of behaviours, as well as physical and emotional signs, include:[19]

- Behaviours: difficulties with workplace relationships, general behaviour changes such as becoming erratic, aggressive, or indecisive, changes to eating patterns; decreased concentration; an increase in errors and difficulties completing tasks
- Physical signs: changes in weight, appearing unkempt, appearing tired
- Emotional signs: irritability, decreased confidence, depression, anxiety, frustration, becoming emotional

It can undoubtedly be difficult to speak with colleagues about their mental health, especially if we have concerns. While it is situation specific, a possible framework may include:[19]

- Finding a quiet time where there is time to talk without feeling hurried
- Finding a quiet space where conversations will not be disturbed
- Asking initially how our colleague is feeling at the moment
- Potentially saying that we have noticed that they have been arriving late at work, or seem to be speaking less than usual
- Giving our colleague the time to answer, and listening empathetically to how they say they are feeling
- Helping them to create a plan for a solution, which might include helping them with accessing services or other resources that may be online
- Creating a timeframe to speak again, to see how they are progressing, such as in two weeks' time.

Compassion fatigue may present in ways that are similar to burnout – and again, being able to recognise these signs and symptoms, to enable the required encouragement and space for recovery, is a critical first step. Symptoms of compassion fatigue may not present until months after a crisis has been endured and then has passed. It may therefore be helpful to have a higher index of suspicion, or a higher sensitivity, to spotting these signs and symptoms in these timeframes. As was stated earlier, for us, as carers, to suddenly feel a 'don't care anymore' attitude can lead to a complex and confusing range of feelings, from distress and fear to worries about not recognising ourselves.

Various strategies can help with recovering from compassion fatigue. If possible, it is helpful to re-designate parts of the workload for a period of time, to decrease exposure to the situation that led to the compassion fatigue. A period of time off work, if possible, is also useful. Time spent away from the necessity to provide care to others can be important in recovery. Similarly, normalising and accepting the feelings of compassion fatigue – even though they can be confusing and even scary – is key. Encouraging conversations around compassion fatigue may also help. These conversations could be talking with a supervisor, a counsellor, occupational health services, a therapist, a colleague, or a friend.

There is a broad range of self-care strategies, and employing a personalised selection of these may help protect against burnout.

Self-care, such as meditation and physical exercise, can help in recovering from compassion fatigue, as in the case with burnout. Journaling and connecting with others may also be useful. It is important to highlight that it may be worth speaking with a GP if we are suffering feelings of not enjoying activities that were previously enjoyable to us. That said, it may also be useful to persevere with these activities, even specifically scheduling them in to encourage us to do them, as it may take time for us to rebalance and redis-cover the joy we previously felt.

Protective factor: Connection

Humans are social creatures, and a lack of connection can have larger impacts on our health and wellbeing than we might initially think. For instance, there is an over 20% increase in the risk of major depressive disorder onset after life events involving social rejection.[20]

As clinicians, we may spend all day seeing patients. Connecting through our work, developing rapport with patients and colleagues, and ensuring that we are part of a well-functioning team is important for effective and efficient delivery of good quality clinical care. In connecting with our work colleagues, we may also be better positioned to help them if we notice changes in their health, as well as to help provide them with protective factors. We may be more likely to confide in and discuss our concerns with each other. We may feel more able to advise our colleagues if it appears they need some time off, or if they need to seek help.

Formal team building exercises are frequently scheduled for us at certain times in our career. At other times, induction processes serve in their place. However, less formal connection is also important. Conversations over a hot drink in a canteen can help us connect in a way that improves our profes-sional connections, as well as our mental health.

It is also important to ensure we are connecting with friends, family mem-bers, and colleagues in an informal, non-work-related way, too. If we feel we don't have time to do this in person, there are various online teleconferencing facilities we can use for video-calls at no cost.

Despite imposed periods of social isolation for much of the community during the COVID-19 pandemic, many doctors and other healthcare practi-tioners have still been required to go to work. This may have led to another layer of conflict around aspects of connection. While seeing our work col-leagues may have actually been theoretically protective for us in some way in spite of physically distancing from colleagues and patients, we may have struggled with thoughts of the risk of 'taking home the virus' as well as our own personal exposure to it. For some, this even meant needing to isolate from vulnerable members of our own household at home.

Protective factor: Access to support

If we feel we need some more support, initially speaking with trusted friends, relatives or colleagues is a suitable first step. If, for whatever reason, we do not feel that this is the right step for us, there are many other avenues of

Chapter 5

support available. Speaking with our GP may be a suitable first point of contact to discuss our concerns about our health, although some of us may be reluctant to do this. As a point to remember, in the UK, part of the compliance requirements for maintaining full registration and a licence to practise with the GMC is to be registered with our own local doctor.

Online, there is a wide range of support groups and charities that can be easily accessed.

United Kingdom based websites include:

- www.mind.org.uk – Mind
- www.sane.org.uk – Sane
- www.headstogether.org.uk – Heads Together

For instances where you need urgent help, the Samaritans free-call number 116 123 is available 24 hours every day of the year.

Other organisations offer support specifically for doctors, nurses, dentists, and other health professionals. These include:

- www.dsn.org.uk – Doctors' Support Network
- www.dochealth.org.uk – where doctors may self-refer for support
- www.rmbf.org – Royal Medical Benevolent Fund
- www.bddg.org – British Doctors and Dentists group for recovering addicts.

Australia based websites include:

- www.lifeline.org.au – Lifeline
- www.beyondblue.org.au – Beyond Blue
- www.headspace.org.au – Headspace mental health
- www.blackdoginstitute.org.au – The Black Dog Institute
- www.headtohealth.gov.au – Head to Health.

Urgent help is available on the 24 hour crisis support line from lifeline, and is available on 13 11 14. Online chat and text services are also available. In an emergency, call 000.

Resources that offer support that is specifically for healthcare practitioners include:

- www.drs4drs.com.au – Drs 4 Drs, with a 24/7 helpline
- www.nmsupport.org.au – Nurse and midwife support, also with a 24/7 confidential support line
- https://www.blackdoginstitute.org.au/ten/ – TEN is 'the essential network' for healthcare professionals.

Resources based in the United States of America include:

- https://suicidepreventionlifeline.org – National Suicide Prevention Lifeline
- www.samhsa.gov/find-help/national-helpline – Substance Abuse and Mental Health Administration
- https://afsp.org – American Foundation for suicide prevention, with 741741 text 'HELLO' crisis text line
- https://www.nami.org National Alliance on Mental Illness.

The National Suicide Prevention Lifeline offers free and confidential crisis support. For emergency assistance, dial 911.

Specifically focusing on the needs of healthcare professionals, there are resources such as:

- https://afsp.org/healthcare-professional-burnout-depression-and-suicide-prevention/ – American Foundation for suicide prevention resource for healthcare professionals
- https://www.amsa.org/ – American Medical Students Association
- https://www.aamc.org/ – Association of American Medical Colleges
- https://www.nursingworld.org – American Nurses Association.

As previously discussed, we have agreed to adhere to a code of professionalism. Under this code, we agree to take steps to ensure that any ill health – be it mental or physical – does not impact on our patients or our ability to deliver quality care.

Some workplaces are leaning towards the inclusion of workplace wellbeing leads. These may be staff members who are identified by a specifically coloured lanyard (such as green) who can be approached about wellbeing initiatives. They may also be available to help with organising team meals or tea-room breaks.

Occupational health departments are usually equipped to help with the diagnosis and treatment of conditions such as burnout. They may be able to assist with managing workplace stress if connection with them is made earlier, rather than waiting until burnout ensues. They may be able to help with aspects such as advice during stressful periods or periods of sick leave, advising of additional appropriate services and advising on 'return to work' schedules.

Speaking with spiritual or religious leaders, including chaplains, may also be of help. If you are involved in a local church or religious group, ensuring you maintain this connection despite a busy working schedule can help with enabling mental health balance and wellbeing.

Our professional bodies advise us to make sure our patients are our primary concern. Yet we need to recognise that if we are impaired, by hunger, tiredness, stress, or a range of other factors, we are not in a position to be able to deliver the level of care that our patients, healthcare system, colleagues and healthcare system requires of us. We need to ensure that we are mindful and alert to the implications of our own health and wellbeing, and that if these are strained or depleted, so may be our treatment of our patients. We need to recognise that taking steps to actively protect and promote our own health and wellbeing not only aligns with the healthcare codes: it is specifically required by them.

NHS Practitioner Health is a UK service that has been set up specifically to act as a free and confidential service to help clinicians – particularly dentists and doctors – with mental health issues.[21] It guarantees confidentiality, aiming to improve accessibility to mental health services that can address the specific needs of clinicians. It also offers an online consultation service. Treatments may also be offered as required, including telephone-based, computer-based, supported and face-to-face Cognitive Behavioural Therapy (CBT).[22]

Protective factor: Judicious use of standardised processes and templates

While healthcare is highly personal, at times the use of technology and templates is of enormous benefit. Research has shown that the use of a template for instances such as in handovers is of benefit. Templates for handovers are key in maintaining clinical effectiveness and safety, given how important a thorough, efficient handover is, and that, by definition, they occur at the end of one clinician's shift and at the start of the next one. By definition, too, one party may be tired, especially after a night shift. The use of a standardised and structured guideline-based handover, in template format, has been shown to:

- Improve compliance
- Improve care quality
- Improve patient safety.[23]

There is a broad range of data which is collected, yet not utilised in any useful way to improve outcomes. More emphasis is now being placed on collecting and using data in an effective and efficient way. Notably during the COVID-19 pandemic, the ability to track symptoms and trace contacts enabled an extra layer of information to be applied to treatment and control efforts. Standardising the way some clinical data is collected may lead to datasets that are able to be used more effectively to improve future clinical outcomes.

Protective factor: Practising self-awareness and meditation/mindfulness

Self-awareness is defined as the '*ability to combine self-knowledge and a dual-awareness of both his or her own subjective experience and the needs of the patient*'.[11] Research shows this may be a critical factor in how people function in times of stress at work or in their personal lives.[11] There is also evidence that increased self-awareness leads to a range of benefits, including improved engagement at work, higher levels of compassion satisfaction, increased self-care – and importantly, improved patient care.[11] Conversely, lower self-awareness levels are associated with higher levels of both burnout and compassion fatigue.

As we will cover later in greater depth, mindfulness meditation helps promote self-awareness, as may practices such as reflective writing. Evidence indicates that mindfulness meditation and reflective writing can lead to a range of benefits such as increasing empathy and decreasing anxiety.[11]

Evidence supports that meditation is of benefit for both physical and mental health conditions, in addition to its potential for increasing self-awareness. Mediation is thought to have originated in India and is generally used these days to refer to a range of different techniques. These different techniques may include:

- Concentrating on physical sensations
- Contemplating
- Listening to nature sounds
- Guided meditations
- Visualising
- Moving with tai chi or yoga poses
- Repetition of a sound or mantra
- Focusing on breathing.[24]

Evidence shows that meditation, and particularly mindfulness, may decrease aspects of psychological stress.[25] Mindfulness also promotes other health benefits, including:[24]

- A decrease in stress.[26]
- A decrease in anxiety.[27]
- A decrease in depression.[28]
- A decrease in pain.[29]
- An increase in memory.[30]
- An increase in efficiency.[31]
- A decrease in blood pressure.[32]

- A decrease in cortisol levels.[33]
- An increase in vagal modulation.[34]

It is thought that some of the effects of meditation may be due to changes in blood flow in the brain, such as increasing the flow to occipital and frontal regions.[35] Some studies even suggest that meditation even affects the physiological parameters we use to measure age.[36] Evidence must be assessed on its own merits as not all studies are of equal quality, but it is interesting to reflect on the wide range of positive impacts potentially associated with practising meditation.

Mindfulness is a specific type of meditation, and a type that has relatively more evidence around its benefits than other types may have. Mindfulness is basically:

- Paying attention
- To the present
- Non-judgementally
- On purpose.[37]

Mindfulness based stress reduction (MBSR) programmes have an evidence base that supports their use in conditions such as generalised anxiety disorder.[38] They may help with a range of physical and mental issues, including ruminative thinking, stress reduction, and trait anxiety in healthy individuals.[39] Essentially, MBSR is a structured programme based on mindfulness, and includes informal meditation, formal meditation, and yoga. The formal meditation components include aspects such as body scans, focusing on breathing, walking meditation, eating meditation, monitoring experiences in the moment, and shifting attention to the senses. Informal meditation components include moments of attention shifting to the present. Yoga practice may include hatha yoga.[40]

Mindfulness based cognitive therapy (MBCT) is designed for helping improve thoughts linked with depression, and has similarities with MBSR.[41] While Cognitive Behavioural Therapy (CBT) targets dysfunctional thoughts and then understanding or modifying them, MBCT aims to simply become more aware of bodily sensations, feelings, and thoughts.[42]

Protective factor: Adequate sleep

Having briefly covered problems around lack of sleep, how can we best promote an adequate quantity of high quality sleep? And given that aspects of healthcare may present organisational barriers to our sleep – such as stress and night shifts – the steps that we take to protect against this, and to promote good sleep, may be even more necessary for healthcare professionals. General sleep hygiene promotes and protects good quality sleep. While the constant changing of rosters means these steps are more challenging, it is advisable to include them where possible in your sleeping arrangements.

Small, basic sleep hygiene steps may lead to significant improvements in overall sleep quantity and quality.

Sleep is a complex process, consisting of stages, that we cycle through in the night. It is generally easier for our body to wake up at the same time each day. This includes weekends. Waking at the same time each day promotes the natural actions of the circadian rhythms – the biological clock regulating when we are awake and when we asleep. However, when we are on night shifts it is more complicated, as we are going to sleep at the time we would normally be waking. In many hospitals, however, it is usually possible to have at least periods with a stable waking time.

While our phones can be a great help in some settings, helping us access accurate medication doses or contact colleagues for additional opinions or advice, they can also be an obstacle to sleep for various neuroscientific reasons. The wavelength of light emitted by them, and by our computers and laptops, too, can have an impact on the production of our sleep hormones, such as melatonin. Natural waves of increasing amounts of these hormones are required for the initiation of sleep. Even exposure to standard room lighting has been shown to affect melatonin production, shortening its duration by approximately 90 minutes and delaying its onset in 99% of subjects in a study of healthy people, when compared to dim lighting exposure.[43] And blue light – the wavelength commonly emitted from phones – tends to have an even greater impact on this.

Therefore, it is a good idea to adjust phone and computer settings to decrease the blue wavelengths in their display at night. Most devices have an automatic setting which will cut this wavelength at specified times. It may be particularly beneficial to decrease the blue wavelength 1.5–2 hours prior to anticipated sleep, since there is an approximately 90 minute delay in the effect.

Addiction cycles that are reinforced in our neurocircuitry via excessive use of social media can also promote wakefulness in the brain. Many social media platforms are devised and designed in such a way as to trigger dopamine spikes. For instance, a 'like' can lead to this, giving us a feeling of pleasure as our reward system is activated. When these are timed at irregular intervals, known as a *random reward schedule*, they become more addictive. This is one of the basic premises behind why slot machines for gambling are so addictive – the gamer never knows when the next 'reward' will come, and so keeps on playing. Content that we read on our phone may also be stimulating and awakening. Even a quick check of our phone near bedtime may stimulate aspects of our brain, which may then keep us awake longer – even leading to a craving in some people for their next 'hit'.

Caffeine is an adenosine antagonist.[44] When present in the body, caffeine connects to receptors that adenosine would normally attach to, effectively blocking the body from recognising the levels of adenosine present. Caffeine, through binding to these receptors, impacts on brain functions, such as memory and sleep. Adenosine receptors have a key role in regulating our sleep.[45] Increasing levels of adenosine lead to increasing levels of sleepiness, while the reverse is true, too. Therefore, part of the effect of caffeine in keeping us awake is that it blocks the natural ways for our brain to realise we are sleepy. It is also important to keep in mind that caffeine remains in our bodies longer than many people realise. In a healthy average adult, the half-life (the time taken for 50% of it to be cleared from the body) of caffeine is approximately 5 hours.[46] By this timeframe, it takes over a day to completely remove a dose of caffeine from our body. Other factors may affect this rate, for example, smoking may increase the rate at which it is cleared, while pregnancy may decrease it. Therefore, given its potential to impact on our sleep, it is advisable to stop drinking caffeinated drinks six hours before our anticipated bedtime.

Napping, luckily, counts towards our total number of sleep hours. Naps are a vital part of night shifts. Shorter naps of 5–15 minutes provide benefits lasting a short period of time, such as 1–3 hours.[47] Longer naps, greater than 30 minutes, improve aspects such as cognitive performance for longer periods; however, sleep inertia on waking may cause initial brief impairment. Research suggests that even short naps of 10 minutes increase alertness. Interestingly, it seems that people who nap more often tend to receive greater benefits from napping than those who nap less often, although many factors are involved, and the whole issue of sleep is not yet fully understood. Evidence indicates that napping leads to less efficient sleep at night.[48] However, during night shifts, given that we know we will suffer from inefficient sleep anyway, naps can be an effective way of gaining some sleep and the associated benefits.

Interestingly, morning sunlight has more blue light wavelengths in it than afternoon light does. Accordingly, if it is a bright morning after a night shift, and we are heading home to sleep, it may help to wear sunglasses to decrease our exposure to the increased blue light. And an eye mask is useful for sleeping when on-call at night if the on-call room is bright, and when sleeping later in the morning after night shifts if there are not blackout blinds.

It is worth remembering that regular physical activity is important for good quality sleep, even though it may be difficult to include during busy clinical placements. Regular physical activity acts by increasing the duration of deep sleep, which is physically restorative. However, it is important to not perform vigorous exercise close to bedtime. Hormones, such as cortisol, required for strenuous workouts, are not conducive to sleep initiation and maintenance and may delay the onset of sleep.

We can promote sleep by the environment that we are in –noise, light, and temperature levels all have an impact. Exposure to heat during sleep has been shown to increase wakefulness, as well as decrease rapid eye movement sleep and slow wave sleep, while exposure to cold, within reason, does not seem to.[49] If our bedroom, or on-call room, is a little cooler, rather than warmer, is can help. A warm shower or bath may help with sleeping; however, if too hot it may have the opposite effect.

After a long day – or night – in a busy clinical environment, it can be difficult to fall asleep. Reaching for a sleeping tablet or sedative may at times be tempting. However, even when used on a short-term basis, these, like other medications, can have harmful side-effects. As previously discussed, dependence and tolerance lead to issues that are more complex to solve. The medications may have a hang-over effect, for instance a benzodiazepine that is too long acting – and this can lead to impairment and cognitive delays the following shift. Furthermore, many of these medications change the complex and cyclical sleep architecture, resulting in an inferior quality sleep compared to natural sleep. While these medications do have a role in some cases, as with all medications, they should not be self-prescribed and should be avoided where possible.

It is useful to bear in mind that changes in our sleep patterns without obvious reasons are potentially indicative of the state of our mental health. Research suggests strong links between depression and sleep – with approximately 70% of people with depression reporting insomnia, and, in younger populations, 40% reporting hypersomnia.[50]

Protective factor: Balanced diet

Many hospitals have cafes and canteens; however, these are often not open during long day or night shifts. Even when they are open, the actual practicalities of getting to them can seem insurmountable some days.

Glucose is the main, preferred source of energy for our brain. It is obtained from different food groups and is a breakdown product that is then used by the brain, muscles, and other organs as energy for functioning. It is notable that research shows that intense periods of concentration and cognitive processes leads to decreases in circulating levels of blood sugar, as measured by peripheral blood glucose.[51] Glucose ingestion enhances performance in certain cognitive tasks such as memory.[52] So, it is logical that low blood sugar (hypoglycaemia) affects our executive cognitive functions – with these including our ability to prioritise, time manage, and organise our thoughts.[53] Given that hypoglycaemia impacts on most of the high-level functions we need and use, it is likely that it also impacts on clinical outcomes and patient care, as well as on our own wellbeing. Therefore, it is logical that we should protect ourselves from hypoglycaemia, particularly since this can be done with a balanced diet.

Most of us, as clinicians, have observed the impact of low blood sugar on patients – for instance, on someone with diabetes.

> *A patient arrives in A&E appearing confused. Along with other investigations, we would take a blood sugar reading. If this reading is low, we could consider this as a possible factor in her confusion.*

Despite seeing the impact that a low blood sugar can have on a patient, we may still not recognise our own symptoms of low blood sugar, especially when we are dealing with this state frequently, as many of us are. Our bodies are extremely capable of balancing our blood sugar requirements, so we, ourselves, may not experience large, pathological shifts in blood glucose levels and more clearly defined associated symptoms. However, starting to feel irritable or sweaty may be a sign of low blood sugar, as may cloudy thinking or headaches.

Low blood glucose levels may make us feel that reaching for a sugary or chocolatey snack is a good solution. This may solve our short-term problem and boost our blood sugars quickly, but we are potentially going to be dealing with an even larger blood sugar crash shortly after. One way that we may be able to help our body achieve a more even blood sugar profile may be through choosing to consume foods that have a lower glycaemic index (GI). Basically, foods that are easily and quickly broken down into sugars in our blood are termed *high GI*. These foods may cause a compensatory spike in insulin, therefore leading to a swift reduction in the blood sugar levels again. Foods with a lower GI generally have their sugars released into the blood stream more slowly. They therefore are less likely to cause a sudden increase in insulin and a corresponding sudden decrease in blood sugar levels. The evidence supporting whether low GI diets are useful for cognitive function is mixed; however, it may be useful in adults.[54]

Simple additions can be made to our diets to include lower glycaemic index foods. Examples of lower GI foods include:

- Apples with their skin on
- Wholegrain pasta
- Oatmeal
- Peanuts
- Low-fat yoghurt.

Alternatively, examples of higher GI foods include:

- White bread
- Bananas
- Sports drinks
- Honey.

There are a range of factors that impact on how our blood sugar levels respond to certain foods.

Our body's response to insulin may have a role, as this hormone helps to keep blood sugar levels in ranges that are healthy. In simplistic terms, when insulin is secreted in a healthy balance, glucose in the blood is converted into glycogen for storage and later use, therefore decreasing the blood sugar levels. If there is either a poor response to the insulin, or a deficit in the insulin (both of which may obviously occur in conditions such as diabetes), this may lead to less effective metabolism of carbohydrates.[55]

For various reasons, proteins may lower the GI of certain foods. For instance, gluten may slow the pancreatic amylases and therefore act to lower the GI of some types of pasta.[55] The degree of processing may impact on the GI of certain foods. Foods that are boiled may tend to have a lower GI than foods that have been roasted.[56] And foods that are of a smaller particle size, through processes such as being ground, may also generally tend to have a higher GI. Fat may prolong the amount of time that it takes for food to travel from the stomach to the small intestine. This may influence the GI profile by lowering it, when a food with fat, such as a potato chip (GI 57) is compared to a food with less fat, such as a baked potato (GI 85).[57]

Suggesting that we take our lunchbreaks is both obvious and fairly unhelpful. Most of us are aware that breaks throughout our day will help with our functioning and productivity, and that eating in these breaks is needed. While it is not always practical or safe to suggest these breaks, we could, generally, become better at covering for our colleagues while they go for their breaks, and them cover for us in return. Particularly on days that are quieter, if they occur, we could potentially try to leave earlier if we are covered. However, a little preparation can go a long way with regards to meals. Taking a handful of nuts into the office is usually possible, or a pre-packaged breakfast bar takes only a moment to eat but can have similar energy values to an entire meal.

Protective factor: Adequate hydration

It's not rare to have a shift where we don't actually have time to use the bathroom. However, consequently drinking too little, so that we don't even need to, is clearly not good for our wellbeing. Signs such as oliguria in our patients would elicit concern and treatment; however, when these same signs appear in us, we are almost grateful! Filling a water bottle at the start of the day, and ensuring we drink it all and refill it by lunch, is a positive and simple step to improve our own wellbeing. Recalling that a normal patient who is 'nil by mouth' may have three one litre bags written up, each delivered over 8 hours, reminds us of how much fluid we, ourselves, need in 24 hours, too.

Evidence shows that even a small decrease in our hydration level may impact on us. A study looking at the impact of soccer players not drinking fluid for 90 minutes showed a 5% deterioration in skills, compared to team-mates who drank during the time period.[58] Many of the studies comparing hydration and concentration are in situations quite different to those which many of us work in – such as at extreme exertion, extreme temperatures, or in the military. Some evidence shows that higher levels of dehydration in older populations relates to poorer memory and attention.[59]

We have briefly discussed some of the impacts of caffeine on sleep. Caffeine is also a diuretic, as is already widely recognised. In one study, drinking caffeinated drinks in large quantities (more than 250–300mg, considered as 5–8 cups of tea or 2–3 coffees), where there had been little or no caffeine in the previous days, led to an increase in urine output from a short-term stimulation of this system.[60] The study found, however, that caffeine-tolerance developed in those who drank caffeinated drinks regularly, so the impact of caffeine in these people was decreased. They therefore concluded that drinking caffeine in a 'normal lifestyle' did not support the idea of caffeine being associated with poorer hydration levels.[60]

There is a range of research on the cognitive enhancing properties of caffeine. This research shows that caffeine, when consumed under conditions of 'suboptimal alertness', may improve memory performance.[61] It may positively affect other areas such as reaction time and in learning passively presented information, but may actually decrease performance when working memory is heavily relied upon.[61]

Protective factor: Optimising thinking styles

As we have already mentioned, many high achievers have perfectionistic personality traits. These traits can help us, as clinicians, maintain the high standards expected of us and that we expect of ourselves. However, perfectionism, which can be defined as either a thinking style or a personality trait, is different to having a drive to achieve the best that we can. A healthy degree of perfectionism helps us achieve accomplishments, and drive our ambitions. Unhealthy, also known as neurotic or maladaptive, perfectionism, is where only 'perfect' is acceptable. This type of perfectionism – expecting only perfect from both ourselves and from others – leads to emotional distress, as concluded by a study of perfection, depression, and emotional vulnerability in nurses.[62]

If we continuously expect only perfection, particularly in clinical situations where this is simply not possible, we end up continuously feeling we have failed. It is thought that perfectionism, in this way, is correlated with depression. In many perfectionists, self-worth is based on goal achievement, with depressive symptoms likely to arise when the goals are not met.[63] It is also likely that perfectionists ruminate, a thinking style where mistakes are thought about repeatedly.[64] Rumination is also linked with depression.

It is human to make mistakes. It goes without saying, of course, that some mistakes are indefensible. A quick look at a list of 'never events' is a good reminder of this (Figure 5.5). This list includes surgery on the wrong site or with the wrong prosthesis, certain medication administration errors, as well as general events relating to falls, injuries, and other adverse events.[65]

However, our time, attention, and healthcare resources are finite. It will help our wellbeing to reflect on this and accept it – and to then respect that we have done our best with the resources that we had available to us at the time.

Chapter 5

surgical
wrong site surgery
wrong implant/prosthesis
retained foreign object post procedure

medication
mis-selection of a strong potassium solution
administration of medication by the wrong route
overdose of insulin due to abbreviations or incorrect device
overdose of methotrexate for non-cancer treatment
mis-selection of high strength midazolam during conscious sedation

mental health
failure to install functional collapsible shower or curtain rails

general
falls from poorly restricted windows
chest or neck entrapment in bed rails
transfusion or transplant of ABO-incompatible blood components or organs
misplaced naso- or oro-gastric tubes
scalding of patients
unintentional connection of a patient requiring oxygen to an airflow meter

Figure 5.5 Never events.[66]

Of course, continuing to maintain high standards for ourselves in our clinical settings is imperative. However, it may be helpful to become aware of when it may be acceptable to relax these standards. It may help us to identify when 'good enough' is good enough. This may help us maintain better quality care over longer periods by avoiding burnout and thus avoiding potential errors associated with it. This is not to advocate poorer patient care. It is to suggest that at times, we may be better served accepting that a presentation or written paper may not be as perfect as we would like it to be, but that it is 'good enough'. The idea that something is 'fit for purpose', or good enough for what is required, can free us to relax our standards, decrease our self-criticism, and enable us to potentially find more balance and joy and less self-criticism and stress. Another way might be to accept that we can be excellent, not perfect, in focal points and goals in our lives, and average, or even mediocre, in others.[67] Consciously selecting those areas where we commit effort, and choosing to celebrate achievements, may help.

Being aware that our expectations of perfection in others may also negatively affect them is key, too. As a part of any team, we all wish to feel our contribution is valued. Demanding perfection from others may actually serve to undermine their best efforts and create a sense of failure in them.

Feelings that other people expect us to be perfect can be addressed by spending some time to more realistically assess what is expected of us. It may help to clearly identify areas where improvement is needed. We can then create a step-by-step plan for how this improvement can be gained. Allocating times for informal 'check ins' or progress reports may also help. It also may help for us to consciously prioritise creating an environment where feedback can be both given and valued. In opening up such environments, we can realise what is actually being expected of us and how we are meeting these expectations – and in all likelihood enable the realisation that perfection is not what is actually being demanded or required.

> *We are working on a busy ward and are required to present at a grand round the next day. Our patients are safe, and we have completed everything that we have to do. We haven't left on time all week, and now it looks like we will need to spend hours to make the perfect presentation. But instead, we decide to work on the presentation for a strict time limit, and after this point, go home – even if we feel that it could have included another diagram.*

Our inherent beliefs about our abilities and intelligence has an impact on how we respond to and cope with hardships. If we have a 'growth mindset', we believe our abilities and intelligence can improve, expand, and develop with effort, while if we have a 'fixed mindset', we believe these cannot change with practice.[68] Research supports that a growth mindset may help us be more resilient, with mistakes potentially affecting us less. Evidence shows that with a grown mindset there is less fear of making mistakes, as these when they do occur are opportunities for learning.[69] Shifting our mindset more towards noticing and reflecting on achievements can help. While reflection on areas that have not gone well is key for our continued learning and to prevent errors happening in the future, reflection on the positive achievement of goals is also key. It can help increase our values of self-worth and work-related enjoyment, both of which may help prevent burnout. Rather than disappointment or self-reprimand at a goal that has not been achieved, reflection upon what could have been done better next time may help.

A growth mindset may increase our resilience and may increase openness around learning from mistakes.

We can help our mental health and wellbeing by making an effort to become aware of our thought processes and beginning to change those that are causing us additional stress. If we start to notice we are dwelling on what we see as a failure, as an outcome that was below what we expected, we may be beginning to be caught in a loop of negative or ruminative thinking. Talking therapies such as Cognitive Behavioural Therapy (CBT) may help. An initial step in this process is to realise that we have tendencies, thoughts, and habits that are not helping us – such as unhealthy perfectionistic traits.

According to CBT, our thoughts, feelings, and behaviours are all cognitively interlinked (Figure 5.6).

This can be further explored in a model where our physical feelings, such as our 'heart racing', can be separated from our emotional feelings, such as 'feeling stressed'. Breaking it down in this way, we can start to analyse and understand how these aspects feed into each other to influence what we do and feel (Figure 5.7).

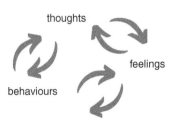

thoughts

feelings

behaviours

Figure 5.6   According to CBT, our thoughts, feelings and behaviours are all interlinked.

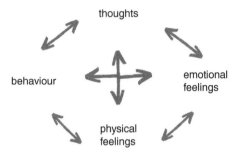

Figure 5.7 Our feelings can be divided into physical and emotional feelings, both of which affect our thoughts and behaviours.

If we want to change how we are feeling, we generally have the power to change either our thoughts or our behaviours, more than our feelings directly. However, changing our thoughts or behaviours can lead to changes in our feelings (Figure 5.8). Once we recognise this, it is easier to elucidate how certain actions or thoughts might lead us to feeling a certain way. Using this model, we can start to reflect on these aspects – and by becoming aware of them, we can learn to change them so that we feel better.

CBT helps us identify some of our unhelpful thinking and behavioural patterns. While beyond the scope of this book, an awareness of some of the techniques of CBT will help us identify automatic thoughts. It can help us to identify thoughts that are unhelpful or not necessarily based on fact, and replace these with thoughts which are more helpful or healthier.[70] Initially, we might try to identify the thoughts we are actually having, and how we are feeling and behaving because of these thoughts. We can then look at more helpful alternatives.

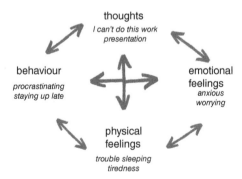

Figure 5.8 Becoming aware of our thoughts, feelings and behaviours can help us to change them.

It is also beneficial to recognise situations that commonly cause us worry, such as:

- Unpredictable situations, where the final outcomes are unclear
- Novel situations, where we don't have any previous experiences to rely on
- Ambiguous situations, where there are multiple different viewpoints or interpretations.[71]

Situations like the recent pandemic are therefore very likely to cause an increase in our worry, given that they satisfy all three of these points, as well as many more. We obviously worry for different reasons. There are also

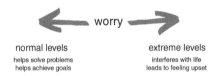

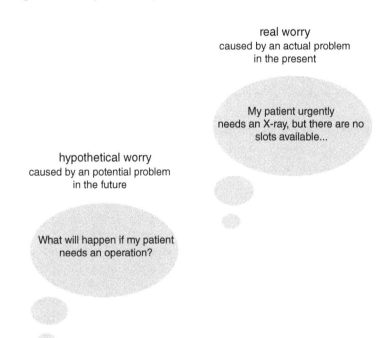

Chapter 5

Figure 5.9 Worry exists on a spectrum.[71]

Figure 5.10 Our worries can be divided into different groups, including real and hypothetical worries.[71]

different types of worry, and being able to identify worries which we can act on helps with our overall sense of wellbeing (Figures 5.9, 5.10).

We do need an element of worry in our lives as this can play a role in keeping us alive. However, excessive worry can lead to a negative impact on our lives. It can decrease our ability to solve problems, potentially increasing errors – and therefore becoming part of a cycle that can cause us more worry.

Things that contribute to us feeling worried can be classed as hypothetical or real. A hypothetical worry is generally not anything we can address, while with a real worry, there may be steps that we can take to help improve the situation we are concerned about.

A decision tree is useful in helping to determine whether a worry is real or hypothetical (Figure 5.11).

Designating a 'worry time' for later in the day helps. As unusual as it sounds, setting aside time specifically for worry may help us to worry less. Giving ourselves a timeslot at the end of the day to list our hypothetical and real worries and to focus on trying to find solutions for them can lead to productive solutions, as well as decreasing the overall level of worry throughout the day.

Developing strategies to help balance unhelpful habits and thought processes takes time. Speaking with a psychologist or psychiatrist may be necessary for some of us. There are a range of different techniques, some of which can be accessed through online programmes, too. This book is not intended to counsel through significant trauma or mental health conditions. It is instead intended to help provide an introduction to some techniques which may help in achieving a more balanced approach to promoting and maintaining mental health and wellbeing.

Protective factor: Appropriate delegation

Learning to delegate and share our workload appropriately is another way that we may be able to help dissipate the effects of perfectionism. As perfectionists, the tendency may be to take on additional work so that we can ensure that it is completely 'perfectly', and that this is under our control. This, however, adds to our own workload and stress, and ironically may mean that the tasks are completed less well due to overload and burnout.

Effective delegation to competent colleagues can help decrease stress and workload, as well as potentially improving the clinical care that is delivered (provided that they, too, are not also over-burdened). Associated with this is the ability to define boundaries and state clearly when we feel that our workload is at risk of becoming too much for us. Being able to say no, or ask for help with the tasks that we need to complete, can help.

It is also key to remember that other people may actually enjoy areas which we do not enjoy. Open conversations about people's preferences often lead to us to realising that this is the case more often than we might initially think.

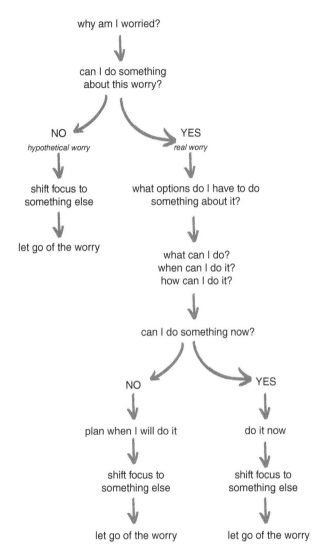

why am I worried?

can I do something
about this worry?

NO
hypothetical worry

YES
real worry

shift focus to
something else

what options do I have to do
something about it?

let go of the worry

what can I do?
when can I do it?
how can I do it?

can I do something now?

NO

YES

plan when I will do it

do it now

shift focus to
something else

shift focus to
something else

let go of the worry

let go of the worry

Figure 5.11   A decision tree can help decide how to manage our worries.[71]

There are several key components of appropriate delegation. These include:

- 'Right task
- Right circumstance

- Right person
- Right supervision
- Right direction and communication'.[72]

While improperly delegating tasks can have a negative impact on clinical care, appropriate delegation should not. To further expand on the above points from a publication on delegation in nursing staff, the 'right task' is one that can be legally delegated and that is also appropriate given the organisation's policies.[73] The 'right circumstances' involve whether or not the appropriate resources, supervision, and equipment are available to carry out the task.[73] The experience, knowledge, training and competencies of the person the task is delegated to need to be understood for them to qualify as the 'right person' – plus the level of supervision available and required also needs consideration, and levels must be met to fulfil 'right supervision'. The requirements around performance, as well as expectations around what needs to be achieved, need to be communicated clearly and directly, as per 'right communication and direction'.[73] Even if a routine task is delegated, it needs to be communicated precisely, with consideration for who takes responsibility for the task results and completion.

Protective factor: Reflection on personal accomplishment

Finding value in what we spend our time at work doing is an important mechanism for our wellbeing. Reflecting on aspects of work that we find rewarding can help shift our biases to help find more of what we find rewarding.

> *Working as a physiotherapist in a busy inner-city hospital, there are often patients waiting for an assessment prior to being discharged. At the end of the day, it sometimes feels as though we have been complained at for being too slow or not seeing as many patients as we 'should' have – and have even being accused of delaying discharges. Instead of focusing on comments such as these, it may help to reflect upon the smile from an elderly gentleman who has just passed his stairs test, or the gratitude of a wife who is pleased to know that her husband can come home safely.*

Reflection on questions such as how much we enjoy talking about our work to others, or if we would continue in our current job if money was no issue, also help us determine how great a sense of personal accomplishment we have.

Protective factor: Physical activity

There is increasing evidence supporting the positive benefits of physical activity on stress reduction and mental and physical health. Most of us know physical exercise is a healthy way to cope with stress. It offers a way for the cocktails of stress hormones to be more in synergy with our physiology. Our 'fight or flight' response provides the means for us to exert physical activity to combat our stress. Therefore, exercise helps us to manage our stresses – both physically and mentally.

There is strong evidence that exercise has a positive impact on a range of physical and mental conditions. A low fitness level is an important predictor of mortality.[74] The evidence shows that we, as clinicians, should encourage activity in our patients in order to decrease their risk of premature death.[74]

We may feel that, at times, there are simply too many items on our 'to do' list, before we can even think about physical activity. The practicalities of a medical career, often meaning leaving home early and/or arriving home late, can lead us to thinking that a simple walk around the block is difficult, as it's too dark, too cold, or too late. Many days it may well be.

There is evidence, however, that as little as 10 minutes of physical activity is of benefit, even at low activity levels.[75] One study found that doing as little as 10–59 minutes of physical activity each week led to an almost 20% reduction in risk for mortality of all causes.[75]

There is strong evidence supporting the positive impacts of physical activity on our mental and physical health.

Another study looked at telomere length to evaluate whether physical exercise affected impacts of chronic psychological stress.[76] They reasoned that stress is involved in many negative physical effects, and so may accelerate cell aging, as measured by the length of the telomere (a region at the end of the chromosome). They predicted that telomere length would be shorter in people under chronic stress, who did not exercise, compared to the telomere length in those who did exercise. Accordingly, they found that in a non-exerciser, a one point increase on the perceived stress scale corresponded to a 15-fold odds increase in the likelihood of the telomere being shorter. By comparison, in an exerciser, the same increase in perceived stress was unrelated to telomere length. They therefore concluded that physical activity provided a buffering effect on the impacts of chronic stress.

Despite being aware of the benefits of exercise, we still often find it difficult to fit in. This may be partly due to stress itself, since evidence shows that experiencing stress actually makes it *more difficult* for us to be active physically.[77]

Since physical exercise does not have to be particularly time consuming or vigorous to deliver benefit, practices such as brief yoga stretches may be easier to squeeze into busy days. Yoga and its associated breathing styles

Chapter 5

has been shown to be helpful support in various conditions, including post-traumatic stress disorder.[78] There are a multitude of free online short work-outs to follow, if we are unsure of which movements to do. A search of Youtube will bring up a large range of instruction videos. Look for ones that have the largest number of views and the highest ratings. Regular stretching exercises, yoga or tai chi are not only helpful in decreasing stress, but they will help protect against poor balance and falls in later life. A small study looking at stress and wellbeing in medical students found that a yoga practice of as little as six weeks improved these parameters.[79]

Even fitting in a few minutes of movement between tasks at work is beneficial. Small things such as making an effort to tense gluteal muscles when getting up from a chair may improve strength and even impact on lower back pain. Ensuring that we maintain correct postures in manual handling movements can also help protect against injury and promote the correct alignment of posture and musculature. If we are unsure of these techniques, many hospitals have access to online courses which we can use to not only refresh our familiarity with correct processes, but also to possibly use for accredited CPD.

Protective factor: Gratitude practices

Gratitude has been found to be linked to wellbeing in multiple studies.[80] Choosing to consciously focus on matters we are thankful for – 'counting our blessings' – benefits us both interpersonally and emotionally.[81] While gratitude may mean different things depending on the context, we are referring here to appreciating and feeling thankful for things which are meaningful to us.

The improvement we feel in our wellbeing from expressing gratitude is due to factors such as positive feelings raised by a sense of thankfulness. Studies have found an association between gratitude and positive aspects such as life satisfaction. For example, a study looking at the impact of a gratitude practice, for example 'counting blessings', found that this group had higher levels of life satisfaction, compared to the control or negative task groups.[82] There is also evidence that gratitude practice positively correlates with perceived sleep duration and quality.[83]

In order to increase our feelings of gratitude, evidence confirms the use of several psychological strategies:

- At the end of the day, or week, writing down three things we are grateful for
- Writing in a journal about areas of our life that we are grateful for
- Sending thank you letters
- Saying 'thank you' during our work shift whenever appropriate
- 'Counting our blessings' and reflecting on things we are grateful for in our life.[80]

Chapter 6 **Protective factors for individual trainee/student implementation**

It is generally harder to break a bad, entrenched habit than it is to start by learning something in a way that forms a good habit. This generalisation holds true in in many areas of life, and health and healthcare are no exception. When commencing our careers, it will pay greater dividends later on if we spend time earlier on considering how we are going to incorporate steps to protect our own wellbeing, and decrease our stress, in our workplace.

We default to our training in times of stress, which is why we spend so long practising emergency drills and the steps in important areas such as basic life support. Hence, it is useful to set up good approaches to stress management as soon as one starts working, so that they are already accessible in times of need.

While 'we don't know what we don't know', we do know that there are several areas where easily preventable errors can be avoided through creating good habits – therefore leading to less stress. So, with a bit of foresight, we can improve our mental health and wellbeing in a two-pronged manner – by improving how we manage our current stress, and aiming to decrease its potential future causes.

The following areas are of key importance in clinicians' careers. Therefore, developing good habits in each of these areas will help us maintain our wellbeing throughout our career. We can 'start as we mean to continue'.

Protective factor: Medical school education styles

As already mentioned, it is easier to start with helpful habits rather than to later have to correct unhelpful ones. Medical school is a key foundation in the healthcare hierarchy so medical school is a good place to start. A survey of medical schools in the USA revealed that almost two thirds of respondents (59%) offered a wellbeing curriculum,[1] covering such issues as:

- Social
- Physical
- Emotional

How to Promote Wellbeing: Practical Steps for Healthcare Practitioners' Mental Health, First Edition. Dr Rachel K. Thomas.
© 2021 Dr Rachel K. Thomas. Published 2021 by John Wiley & Sons Ltd.

- Spiritual
- Financial.[1]

The survey concluded, however, that more evidence was needed on the impact of these curricular changes. Other research has suggested that wellbeing should be included not only within the formal curriculum, but also in the so-called 'hidden' curriculum.[2] It was suggested that this hidden curriculum detracted from efforts to promote aspects of wellness and discouraged help seeking behaviours, and even added to stigma around mental health.[2] It was even suggested that by medical schools being intolerant of absence due to illness, they were in fact adding support to presenteeism in the healthcare system's structure.[2] Wellbeing may not necessarily be improved by adding more wellbeing activities to already-full curricula. This may actually become counter-productive, adding more stress and lengthening already long 'to-do' lists for students.

There is, of course, a requirement to enable students to develop skills to handle stress, given it is unavoidable in clinical practice. However, research suggests that producing cohorts of students who cope well with educationally stressful curricula may not be effective in promoting resilience against work stresses. The current curricula may inadvertently be promoting mental health conditions, stress, and burnout, rather than resilience.[2]

The medical school environment – and indeed that of any healthcare practitioner's training – needs to become one where wellbeing habits and self-care habits are effectively taught, so that future careers can be built on resilient mental health and wellbeing foundations, in order that we can focus on providing optimal care for patients.[2] Medical school should provide an environment where taking steps to optimise our ability to keep ourselves healthy is championed and respected.

We can readily recall the stress and pressure we felt around examinations. The necessity to get 'good grades' meant we spent hours not only studying, but stressing as well. Interestingly, research on examination grading has shown that using a pass/fail method, rather than letter-grading, led to improvements in the students' feelings of satisfaction and wellbeing.[3] While this may intuitively make sense, this research, perhaps counter-intuitively, also found that this was not at the cost of reducing their attendance performances, residency placements, or test scores.[3]

Protective factor: Good habits around maintaining patient confidentiality

We need to develop effective practice in maintaining patient confidentiality early on, as it is obviously of core importance in healthcare. Simple steps to take can be ensuring that we do not discuss patients in common areas such as hospital cafeterias or elevators, where we may be overheard. Even if we are discussing a different patient, if someone hears us and recognises us as someone on the team looking after them or their loved one, it may be natural for them to assume that we are talking about them or their relative. A poor prognosis we may be discussing for someone else suddenly becomes, in their eyes, their problem, and will cause the patient unwarranted stress.

When we are concerned about a patient and have an opportunity to discuss their case, it is best to use patient initials, rather than names, since it is not always possible to find somewhere private for discussion without the possibility of being overheard. Using bed numbers as an identifier is not advisable as it depersonalises the patient, and bed changes lead to confusion.

It is best to start creating good habits around safe storage and disposal of sensitive information. Most hospitals have clearly signed confidential waste bins. Consider writing jobs lists in a book that can be closed, rather than on a page which may be seen by other patients during ward rounds. Any transporting of patient lists, as well as emails with patient details, needs to be carried out in a secure manner.

Lapses in confidentiality can lead to significant stress and concern – for our patients as well as for us.

There are associated stresses for both the patient and us, if confidentiality is accidentally breached. Breaching confidentiality can lead to the patient losing faith in us and our team, and may also lead to disciplinary action. This then adds to our stress, as well as potentially negatively impacting our future. In such cases, it may be advisable to speak with our superiors, and even the external support bodies providing insurance or indemnity, as soon as possible.

Protective factor: Maintaining thorough record keeping

Fastidious record keeping is another habit which is easier to develop earlier, rather than later, in our careers. Most hospitals are now moving to a digital system, but some still use hand-written records. We should ensure that any writing we do is in black pen, legible, and as complete as possible. It is easy to forget that patient notes are legal documents. All patient entries need to be dated and signed, and we are responsible for anything that we record. We have to ensure that we do not write anything we wouldn't be prepared to have read out in court.

Ensuring that our record keeping is thorough is not only good practice for optimal patient care; it can also help decrease our stress in other ways, too. For instance, while it may be more time-consuming initially to write thorough patient notes, it can save time in the long run. Having more substantial, accurate records can decrease our workload by making it easier for other teams to contribute optimally to the care, leading to better patient outcomes.

One of the patients on our ward has developed a skin rash, and we have requested a dermatology review. Having clear, succinct and accurate notes on the patient will assist the reviewing team to contribute as effectively as possible to the patient's care. If our notes are illegible or not as thorough as required, we will inevitably be bleeped, and interrupted from other work, in order to fill the reviewing team in on the patient. While conversations between teams are, of course, beneficial, if it is only to clarify what is going on with the patient, when thorough notes would have sufficed, it is a drain on both our time and theirs.

Protective factor: Maintaining clear communication

Good communication skills are a key part of being a clinician. There are three core components, as most of us are aware, in face-to-face communication, which many patient-related encounters are:

- Words
- Voice tone
- Non-verbal behaviour.[4]

According to research, words are responsible for only 7% of our communication, our tone of voice for 38%, and it is our non-verbal behaviour that is responsible for over half of our communication, (55%).[4] It sounds obvious, but we may not often consider that, as our non-verbal communication is by definition non-verbal, we are already starting to communicate long before we open our mouths. The way we approach a patient is communication, as is the way we maintain eye contact and how we hold our head. Classically, we receive training in communication as clinicians – appropriate ways to start difficult conversations, use of open-ended questions, jargon-free language, and so forth. However, we receive less training in non-verbal communication, and given its importance, it may be useful to reflect on it and consider ways to improve it.

Effective non-verbal communication impacts positively on patient outcomes. Research supports that when we use non-verbal communication appropriately, we convey our feelings of empathy, while if we use it inappropriately, we may, instead, only convey feelings of disinterest.[5]

Non-verbal behaviours that lead to patients feeling more satisfied include:

- Nodding
- Leaning forward
- Increasing eye contact
- Decreasing interpersonal distance.[6]

It is key to remember that increasing any of these excessively tends to have the opposite effect – over-enthusiastic efforts to build rapport tend to be seen as insincere. Behaviour can be difficult to modify authentically, but it is important to at least be aware of the significance of non-verbal communication.

Current guidelines relating to the use of PPE may impact on our ability to communicate in some ways, particularly our non-verbal communication. Patients may no longer be able to see a smile, as it is obscured by a mask. However, it is important to still smile in greeting, since a smile impacts on the rest of our communication and on other areas of our face, such as our eyes. And patients that may lip read to facilitate understanding will not be able to do so if a mask is in the way, meaning other communication support may be required.

It is important to remember to update patients as soon as possible on investigation result timeframes, as well as the results themselves. If there are reporting delays, quickly mention this to the patient as it can save them from worrying unnecessarily. They may understandably start to worry that a delayed result automatically means a 'bad' result.

Protective factor: Planning training requirements

Ensuring that educational programmes and obligatory supervisory reports are completed in time for our progress through training is obviously key. These can be a great source of stress if they are left to the last minute.

It is advisable to become familiar with the signoffs and workplace-based assessments required at the start of each new rotation or education module. Committing to a feasible plan of a number of these each month means we aren't left at the end of the period chasing signatures, when we should be focussed on our patients and possibly other examinations.

With planning, we can decrease a workload that we might otherwise be adding to through accidental duplication. Many of the requirements that need to be met can be covered with work we are doing anyway, and a bit of lateral thought. Being familiar with this early on means we can keep our eyes out for routine processes and procedures that we are doing which can be used simultaneously as signoffs.

If we are required to have supervised sign-offs for activities such as cannulation, aim to do this on quiet afternoons when our colleagues have time, and send through sign-off forms promptly. Completing these activities when the wards permit, rather than when a deadline looms, will lead to less stress for us, and likely better outcomes - for both us and the patient.

Chapter 7 **Emergencies in mental health and wellbeing**

Part of being human means that we will all have the occasional time when we feel we cannot cope – irrespective of whether we work as a clinician or not.

Doctors are more reluctant to access support services when they need them, compared to the wider community. Evidence has shown that there are many reasons why people avoid seeking medical care. They may perceive that they are a low risk for the need for medical intervention, may have barriers in the way of accessing care, or they may perceive aspects of care as negative.[1]

Reasons for people avoiding seeking help include:

- A perception that the condition will get better
- A perception that the condition is not too bad
- Lack of insight into own health
- A perception that there is not enough time to seek help
- Long wait times to get an appointment
- A concern about health conditions being documented.

While any or all of these reasons may contribute to a delay in clinicians seeking assistance, they may also have particular fears concerning how a mental health diagnosis may impact career progression. Establishing clear frameworks of potential pathways for professional and personal emergencies may help improve access.

Professional emergency: Pandemics

The COVID-19 crisis is unlike any other that we, or our hospitals, have experienced in recent times. It has the potential to leave long-lasting damage on the clinicians within it, even once the acute waves of illness have passed. Evidence suggests that the likelihood of us developing psychological injury is

How to Promote Wellbeing: Practical Steps for Healthcare Practitioners' Mental Health,
First Edition. Dr Rachel K. Thomas.
© 2021 Dr Rachel K. Thomas. Published 2021 by John Wiley & Sons Ltd.

dependent on how well we are supported 'before, during, and after a chal-lenging incident'.[2] Support strategies for helping to manage the impacts of a crisis include.[2]

Before and during the crisis:

- Preparing staff for what they will be exposed to, and what they will have to deal with, in advance of their exposure will help decrease the stresses they will face. An objective assessment of the issues may be difficult to define but will be helpful in the longer term
- Preparing staff for decisions that may be morally challenging, such as how to allocate limited healthcare resources
- The use of reflective practice for discussions may be helpful
- Access to trained professionals for members of staff who feel particularly distressed
- Developing and including support processes as part of the routine
- Developing and including education around the causes, signs, and symp-toms of mental health concerns, as well as those for moral injury
- Ensuring that both junior and senior staff are actively monitored for men-tal health and wellbeing.

After the crisis has passed:

- NICE guidelines advise 'active monitoring' of personnel to enable early identification of anyone who has been negatively affected to the stage of becoming unwell. These people can be encouraged to access suitable care
- Encouraging and promoting allocated time to reflect on the crisis, in order to create a narrative promoting personal growth and meaning, rather than one concentrating on the trauma
- For the clinicians who are caring for colleagues affected by moral injury, it is important to remember that we tend to avoid talking about moral injury, due to feelings such as shame. This tendency may lead to poorer therapeu-tic outcomes.

Professional emergency: Patient mental health

Mental health – as with physical health – is affected by many factors, and we never know when we may be presented with a sudden, acute deterioration of a patient. As with any area of medicine, an acute deterioration in mental health can be alarming – for both the patient and the clinician – particularly when it is the first such occurrence they have experienced.

Chapter 7

Many hospitals have an on-call Psychiatry team to contact in such an instance. As with any medical specialty, these teams expect to be contacted when a colleague needs help with a patient's condition, and we should have a low threshold for contacting them when necessary. Usually this is done by requesting the on-call Psychiatry Consultant or Registrar through the hospital's main switchboard.

In the community, when we have concerns over a patient's mental health, a referral to mental health services may be appropriate. Services such as Improving Access to Psychological Therapies (IAPT) facilitate access to CBT. However, if we are seriously concerned with an acute situation, calling ambulance services may be necessary.

A framework which Psychiatrists follow includes one for evaluating risk. This risk assessment is based on factors including, but not limited to:

- Risk to self, such as self-harm, self-neglect
- Risk to others, such as through violent outbursts
- Risk to reputation, such as through actions stemming from low insight
- Risk to finances, such as compulsive over-spending.[3]

A broad range of first line interventions may be appropriate to use, depending on the situation and possibly including both behavioural and pharmacological treatments.

Acutely unwell patients can be sectioned under various Mental Health Acts, allowing them to be detained or treated against their will where this is in their best interest.

Professional emergency: Whistleblowing

'Whistleblowing' has been recognised as being important for improving patient safety, despite it having a complicated past in institutions such as the NHS in the United Kingdom. Many clinicians may be fearful of the concept of 'Whistleblowing'. Feeling the need for whistleblowing an incident or person can increase our stress and take a significant toll on our wellbeing. However, understanding that whistleblowing may be a part of our professional obligations, and one that it important ultimately for patient wellbeing, may help.

A whistleblower is someone who reports something extremely concerning in an environment, such as a particular wrongdoing. The term is based on the historical use of whistles by the English police force when a crime was being committed.

There are several common areas where a clinician may consider acting as a whistleblower. These may be concern around:

- A single incident
- An individual over a period
- An entire department
- An entire healthcare system.

Many clinicians are reluctant to act as a whistleblower. For instance, research supports that despite physicians generally being aware of and in support of a professional commitment to report incompetent or otherwise impaired colleagues, many do not report this when actually faced with a relevant situation.[4]

Furthermore, many doctors or clinicians do not inherently trust the systems in place for reporting adverse incidents. A survey of British doctors found that while 97% of over 2,500 survey respondents thought that a reliable reporting system would increase the patient level of care, 80% would not trust such a system run by the Department of Health or their local Healthcare Trust.[5] The vast majority instead felt that an independently run system would be a preferable option.

Our particular clinician obligations may require us to act on incidents such as:

- Unsafe working conditions – including a lack of PPE
- Patient safeguarding failures
- Patient safety concerns
- Inadequate standards of clinical practice, or malpractice
- Inadequate staff training
- Inadequate policies or lack of adherence to policies
- A culture of bullying amongst staff
- Unwell or stressed staff who are unable or unwilling to seek help
- Concerns over medication administration.[6]

Research indicates that the reporting of critical incidents may best be done via electronic reporting means.[7] Many hospitals have Datix, or a similar system, already in place for doing so.

If we do happen to come across any incidents that we find particularly concerning, there are several possible avenues by which to report them.

The National Patient Safety Association (NPSA) was established in 2001 to identify both issues in patient safety and potential solutions.[8] Since 2012, the NPSA has been part of the NHS Commissioning Board Special Health Authority.[9] Errors commonly reported to the NPSA include medicine reconciliations – where the medications that a patient is taking prior to hospital admission are incorrectly identified and therefore incorrectly listed on their admission form.

Chapter 7

Some clinicians fear they may suffer retribution if they highlight or report serious concerns. Many whistleblowing predecessors have subsequently suffered damage to their careers. Steve Bolsin, one of the most prominent whistleblowers in the UK, raised serious concerns about the excessively high paediatric heart surgery death rates in the 1990s in Bristol and as a consequence suffered severe damage to his reputation and career.[10]

If one is seriously concerned, various possible courses of action are available. Initially, the best idea is to try to resolve the issue at a local or trust level. Approaches include:

- Approach a senior clinician
- Approach a senior manager
- A letter to the trust, such as the trust executive
- A letter to the Department of Health
- A letter to the Royal College as appropriate.

Concerns may also be raised through the GMC or other professional regulatory bodies. Prior to raising concerns, it may be helpful to discuss the best course of action with an indemnity body, or even with a lawyer, depending on the situation. Generally, we may need to record aspects such as the date, time, and location of an incident, and who was involved, in a written format for our own records to refer to, as soon after the event as possible. Our recollections change with time, and so doing this as soon as we are able to will help to maintain the accuracy and integrity of our records.

The NHS has a whistleblowing helpline, which can be also accessed anonymously.[11]

Telephone: 08000 724 725 | Web: www.wbhelpline.org.uk | Email: enquiries@wbhelpline.org.uk

And WhistleblowersUK is at https://www.wbuk.org

In the United States, systems such as The National Whistleblowing Centre are available through which complaints can be registered. (see http://www.whistleblowers.org)

In Australia, the Australian Healthcare Practitioners Regulation Agency (AHPRA) regulates healthcare practitioners (see https://www.ahpra.gov.au).

While it can be a stressful situation to be in, it is worth remembering that working as a healthcare practitioner means that we a have a professional code to follow and a duty to follow it. Part of this means putting our patients and their safety first. And given that in some environments there may be a feeling that to criticise our colleague is not good practice, putting patient wellbeing at the forefront of our actions as clinicians is key.

Personal emergency: Personal crisis

If we need urgent help, the Samaritans free-call number 116 123 is available 24 hours of each day of the year.

Practitioner Health Services are at https://www.practitionerhealth.nhs.uk/ and on 0300 0303 300

The British Medical Association has released counselling and peer-support wellbeing services on 0330 123 1245. They have also released a 10-tip plan to help support colleagues and our own wellbeing during crises such as COVID-19:[12]

- The pairing of staff with more experience with those that are newer or less experienced
- Leadership, visibility, and accessibility of senior staff
- Staff role rotation varying between higher stress and lower stress positions
- The use of support groups to open conversations between staff members
- Helping accessibility of breaks for food and drink, as well as encouraging simple activities such as breathing exercises
- Encouraging the use of existing family and friends support networks
- Encouraging access to support networks such as the tools provided by services such as the BMA
- Encouraging the use of proven life-style interventions such as physical activity
- Accepting that feelings of stress or anxiety may be a normal response to what is arguably an abnormally stressful period
- Encouraging an awareness of signs that colleagues may need additional support.[12]

As previously discussed, chatting with a trusted friend, family member, or GP, is a worthwhile way to seek support during a personal crisis. However, if we feel our circumstances are becoming extremely acute, we should not hesitate in contacting ambulance services or even the police.

Chapter 7

Chapter 8 **Mental health and wellbeing toolkit**

This book highlights problem factors, as well as protective factors, currently influencing our mental health and wellbeing as clinicians. It is by no means an exhaustive or conclusive exploration of all factors, but aims to highlight ways to make improvements for our mental health and wellbeing.

This final section provides a summary and brief explanation of potential protective factors as a 'tool kit' to be employed as an aide memoire. This brief refresher of some of the main points can help promote our ability to select a technique easily in a time of need, particularly when we are under time pressure and feeling stressed.

No single approach will work for everyone. In fact, no 'one thing' will work every time, even for the same individual – even if it was helpful in the past.

Sometimes we may think that we just need a 'quick fix' to improve how we are feeling. However, temporary solutions such as reaching for sugary treats or caffeine hits, or even 'zoning out' in front of the television, are not the best answer. It will be more beneficial to our long-term mental wellbeing if we can improve our feelings by actually employing mood-shifting behaviours. Many of these have been discussed at length, and the evidence behind them considered, in the previous pages. The following toolkit forms a quick ready-reference guide for when they are needed.

Behavioural changes can be difficult, and we may often default to unhealthy habits in times of stress. However, implementing some of the suggested ideas in this toolkit may help.

From a behavioural change point of view, we may be better off trying to include one small change for a period of time, before adding another one. Trying to change in many areas at the same time is more likely to be both difficult and unsustainable. It is advisable to select one behaviour from the

How to Promote Wellbeing: Practical Steps for Healthcare Practitioners' Mental Health, First Edition. Dr Rachel K. Thomas.

toolkit, see how it fits into our life and work schedule over a period of weeks, and then evaluate if we feel better for including it. At this point, we can try to decide if we wish to keep putting in the effort for it to become a part of our routine, or if a different version of these wellbeing tools may help us more instead.

Reframing

Trying to change the way a situation, event, or even a feeling, is viewed – basically trying to look at it from a different angle – can help us. It can help us with trying to see something from a different perspective if we come up with different meanings behind something that has left us feeling stressed or down.

Weighing the evidence

If a negative thought is causing us stress, trying to look at the facts that support it can help us test how true it most likely is. We can start to look at what evidence there is to support our worrying thought, and start to challenge its strength. We may find that some of the things we assume to be true may not hold up to scrutiny.

Softening black-and-white thinking

It can be deceptively easy to see things as 'all good', or alternatively 'all bad', particularly when we are feeling down. This way of thinking can actually increase our stress. It is more helpful to realise that things are very rarely 100% 'all or nothing'. Generally both positive and negative aspects are present, and realising this will decrease the stress involved in situations. Trying to regard things as not totally black, nor totally white, but instead as shades of grey, can help.

Focusing on the benefits

It is not possible for us to help everyone. We have limited resources. We can only do the best that we can, with the resources that we are provided with. There will always be some patients that we are unable to help, no matter how hard we try, or what resources we have. Focusing thoughts on patients we have helped, rather than on any we were unable to help, can strengthen our mental wellbeing in times of stress.

Journaling

Spend a few moments at the end of each day writing about the day's activities. This can help us gather information on how we feel about things that have happened in our day, including events or interactions which have led to us feeling stressed on unhappy. Journaling can also provide us with a mechanism for reflection and learning.

Reflecting

As clinicians, we are generally required to reflect formally on events, as part of maintaining our professional licences. The GMC requires medical doctors to do this in a structured way within each yearly appraisal cycle. The time we spend reflecting on cases that went well will build our confidence up. In addition, we can learn from reflection on instances that did not go quite so well and formulate how we can improve outcomes if a similar situation should ever arise again. Reflecting on a common mission and feeling part of our team will also add to our sense of mental wellbeing.

Challenging thought processes

If we believe, for example, that in order to be a good healthcare practitioner, we must never make a mistake or must know everything, then if we do make a mistake or don't know something, even if it may be insignificant, it may lead to us feeling stressed or negative about our work. Instead of blindly accepting this belief, we may spend some time thinking about what actually makes a good clinician. At times we may find that what we think makes a good clinician is in fact different to what a patient actually values in an interaction.

Pausing

It is quite okay to take a break. Trying to 'push on' when we are feeling excessively stressed does not necessarily mean we will do things more quickly or efficiently. Taking a quick break to recharge – even a few minutes outside – gives us the chance to de-stress, and the opportunity to return to the task at hand with fresh vigour.

Delegating

There are usually some aspects of our work which are essential that we do ourselves. However, for times when we are feeling exceptionally 'snowed under', delegating work appropriately to others can relieve stress. Discuss different tasks with our colleagues, particularly those that cause us stress. Delegating with an awareness of what our colleagues enjoy may also mean that we can sometimes delegate work we prefer less to someone else who actually enjoys it more than us – and vice versa.

Working as a team

While we each have our own roles, it is important to remember that we are part of a team and have support from others available. It can help to remind ourselves of this and request support if required. Sharing our experiences can help to normalise how we are feeling, and we might find that we are not the only one who has been feeling this way.

Noticing anticipatory stress

Be aware that often when an event we were stressed about actually happens, we realise 'it wasn't so bad after all'. It is common for the worrying over some future event to be worse than the stress of the event actually happening. Sometimes worrying about something in advance may be useful, in order to help us prepare thoroughly. However, if we get so stuck in a cycle of anticipatory stress over a future event that it weighs excessively on our minds, it may hinder our ability to perform well at all.

Accepting 'good enough'

Realising that, in some situations, such as giving presentations, it is rarely possible to achieve perfection. In these cases, learning to accept 'good enough' may help reduce stress. This does not mean, of course, only checking partially for allergies, or only almost administering medications. It means that sometimes a 'perfect' presentation in a meeting, or being less prepared for speech, might help decrease stress. Spending some time learning to identify where 'good enough' might be satisfactory can also help.

Replacing 'should' and 'must'

Replacing 'should' with 'could', particularly when we are talking to ourselves, can help to give us more options about our behaviour, thoughts, and feelings. Using 'should' and 'must' can lead to us feeling under greater expectations and with more rigid rules around what is acceptable.

Chapter 8

Playing out 'what if. . .?'

If we are concerned about a situation, playing out the possible outcomes helps us with our wellbeing. Imagining through the various outcomes – the good as well as the bad – will help us to allay our fears, since we can obtain a more balanced view of what will most likely happen.

> *E.g. We have a presentation coming up, and hate public speaking. It is a monthly morbidity and mortality meeting, and our colleague who was going to speak has called in sick. It feels like we will stand there with nothing to say. In actual fact, this is pretty unlikely. Similarly, it is pretty unlikely that we will give an Oscar-winning performance. What is more likely is that we will be able to make some relevant comments, and the session will pass.*

Connecting

Try relaxing by allocating a few minutes each day to connecting with friends and family members important to us. In a healthcare setting, we may spend all day around people, yet not actually 'connect' on an interpersonal level with anyone. This could be as little as a phone call, or sitting down together for a coffee on a break. Try to spend a few moments each day speaking with someone about our, or their, interests – anything other than work. If we enjoy speaking about work, this is helpful too; however, expanding our connections beyond this provides us with better life balance. Discussing cases is an easy way to connect with colleagues – just ensure that when discussing cases we maintain patient confidentiality.

Mentoring and buddying-up

We can try to find a suitable colleague for mentoring or buddying in order to help clarify our career pathway, and to handle obstacles along the way. We don't need to wait for formalised programmes of mentoring or buddying: we can start our own. Particularly when starting a new position, having someone who 'knows the ropes' to talk to can help enormously.

Being thankful

Pausing at the end of each day to reflect on things we are grateful for can strengthen mental wellbeing. Searching for what we are grateful for may help us on several levels, including helping our mental filters to 'tune into' even more of what we may be grateful for.

Feeling a sensation

Mindfulness practices can be included anywhere in our day. Each time we manage to include them, we can use this as an anchor to the present. We can do this simply by feeling a sensation, and not judging it, at a moment in our day.

> *E.g. While washing our hands between patients, concentrate on feeling the water – how cool or warm it is, its pressure as it runs out of the tap. Rather than thinking about the previous patient, or worrying about the coming one, try to use this as a mechanism to embed ourselves in the present. In this way, washing our hands can become a small yet effective mindfulness ritual – while ensuring we are maintaining adequate hand hygiene.*

Progressively relaxing our muscles

From time to time, we all are guilty of carrying tensions accumulating during the day around with us. An effective way to relax at night may be to move through our body with progressive muscle relaxation. Starting at one point in our body, say our feet, squeeze momentarily and then fully relax the area that we are focused on. Then move on to the next section of our body, say our calves, and progressively around our whole body. Alternative there are various guided meditations that can be found online to assist with this.

Progressively mentally scanning our body

This is similar to the progressive muscle relaxation. However, instead of tensing and releasing each area that we focus on, simply observe how it is feeling. Is it warm, or is it cool? Can we feel any vibrations or other sensations? Try not to judge whatever we observe: simply observe it and move on to the next body region.

Deep breathing

Our breathing can affect our physiological and emotional state. Simply taking a few slow deep breaths in and out helps to calm and focus us. Similar to increasing our awareness of the act of washing our hands, this can be done between patients as a way to delineate the issues of one patient from the next. Counting the length of the breaths may also help – counting the inhale for four counts, and the exhale for four counts. Increasing the exhale by a count – such as inhaling for 4, then exhaling for 5 – also contributes to a feeling of calmness.

Chapter 8

Focusing on a physical sensation

Try intentionally focusing on one sole detail for a few minutes each day, such as our breathing, a sensation, or a sound. Including basic meditation practices such as mindfulness in our daily routine is a simple ritual that can significantly decrease our stress levels. Mindfully observing our breathing, following each breath as it comes in and out and sitting still to notice this, even for just a few minutes, can be useful. Rhythmically repeating one single sound over and over in our mind is another option, as practised in Vedic meditation.

Moving

Aim to include 10 more minutes of movement every day to improve our mental and physical health and wellbeing. It's easy to increase incidental exercise, by taking the stairs between wards rather than the elevators, or by walking a few extra blocks to get home. All this exercise contributes to increasing our daily activity levels.

Drinking de-caffeinated drinks after 3pm

Cease drinking coffee or other caffeinated drinks by 3pm on a day shift. This will help us to fall asleep more easily at night, since the half-life of caffeine's stimulating effect on the metabolism is 5–6 hours. Be conscious of the fact that healthier alternatives, such as green tea and matcha, may also have contain caffeine. If we are drinking a lot of caffeine, an easy plan to decrease it is to cut out our caffeinated drink of the day and substitute it with a decaffeinated alternative, for several days. Then, when we have established that routine, cut out another one until we are drinking our last one before 3pm.

Removing blue light after 8pm

Set our mobile phone and other tech devices to a 'night shift' setting, so that the blue light and the brightness are automatically decreased at least an hour and a half before we intend to go to sleep.

Prioritising sleep

Aim to prioritise going to sleep, even though at times a box-set or extra television show can be tempting. An extra half hour's sleep here and there adds up.

Starting and keeping to a regular sleep schedule

Where possible have a regular bed-time and wake-time schedule. Try to go to bed at the same time each night when on day shifts. While night shifts may hinder this, providing our body with a predictable daily rhythm contributes positively to our overall wellbeing.

Drinking enough water

Keeping a bottle of water at a desk we access frequently, or committing to drink a bottle before we start our day, will help us stay well-hydrated.

Eating well

Given how busy shifts can be, and the quality of food available in some healthcare systems, it is not surprising that our diets may suffer at times. Simple steps to plan ahead will have big impacts on our mood, concentration, and ultimately even patient care – and on our waistlines. Having a healthy, low GI snack in our bag can help with resisting sugar cravings and with beating hunger. Bags of nuts, apples with their skin on, low fat cheese, boiled eggs and other quick-to-prepare snacks can help decrease the risk of dips in blood sugar, and the associated concentration loss, occurring when we don't have time to find a healthy meal.

Sitting less

Incidental exercise is key in offsetting a sedentary lifestyle. Some even say that 'sitting is the new smoking'. Many healthcare positions already involve being on our feet almost all day. However, for the more sedentary work, including small increases in movement throughout the day can help offset the independent risk factor for health that is due to a sedentary lifestyle. Take the stairs in between wards instead of the elevator at least once each day, if not more often.

Going outside

It may be difficult to find the time to take breaks at times; however, when they are possible, try taking at least one of our breaks outside – in fresh air that has not been through air conditioning, and in light that has not been filtered through windows. A short break outside, even if it involves taking some of the break time to get there, will be more restorative than sitting in a coffee room or hospital café.

Chapter 8

Talking

Start conversations on our mental health. This will help normalise these for others. Speaking up if we are feeling stressed helps not only ourselves, but also could benefit our colleagues who may be in difficulty.

Accessing online resources

NHS – www.nhs.uk – for advice on a range of physical and mental health conditions from the National Health Service.

Mind – www.mind.org.uk – for a range of resources, including information and how to access support, for a range of mental health conditions.

The Samaritans – www.samaritans.org – 24 hours a day, 7 days a week, telephone support for people feeling in crisis.

Practitioner Health – www.practitionerhealth.nhs.uk – An online and telephone service specifically for supporting clinicians.

Beating the Blues – www.beatingtheblues.co.uk – A series of eight modules, each approximately 50 minutes, teaching cognitive and behavioural skills.

Beyond blue – www.beyondblue.org.au – Resources and support to help optimise mental health.

Lifeline – www.lifeline.org.au – Crisis support including a digital lifeline, and groups including bereavement and financial counselling.

Headspace – www.headspace.org.au – Supporting youth mental health through phone and online services, as well as physical locations.

Blackdog Institute – www.Blackdoginstitute.org.au – Tools and resources to support mental health, and a focus on research into mental health across the lifespan.

MoodGYM – www.moodgym.com.au – A series of five modules, each approximately 30–45 minutes, teaching skills such as how to modify negative thoughts, and behavioural activation.

Substance Abuse and Mental Health Administration – www.samhsa. gov – US department of health and human services resource, including a treatment locator

National Alliance on Mental Illness – www.nami.org – resources including a video library and discussion groups, and a help line.

References

Introduction

1 Donaldson, L. (2000) *An Organisation with a Memory: Report of an Expert Group on Learning from Adverse Events in the NHS Chaired by the Chief Medical Officer*: The Stationery Office, London
2 https://www.gmc-uk.org/ethical-guidance/ethical-guidance-for-doctors/good-medical-practice
3 https://www.gmc-uk.org/ethical-guidance/ethical-guidance-for-doctors/goodmedical-practice/duties-of-a-doctor
4 https://www.gmc-uk.org/ethical-guidance/ethical-guidance-for-doctors/goodmedical-practice/domain-2----safety-and-quality#paragraph-28
5 https://www.nmc.org.uk/standards/code/read-the-code-online/
6 https://www.gov.bm/sites/default/files/Standards-of-Practice-for-Allied-Health-Professions-V1-w-cover.pdf

Preface

1 Hare, D. L., Toukhsati, S. R., Johansson, P., & Jaarsma, T. (2014) Depression and cardiovascular disease: a clinical review. *Eur Heart J*. Jun 1;35(21):1365-72. doi: 10.1093/eurheartj/eht462. Epub 2013 Nov 25.

Chapter 1

1 World Health Organization. The Global Burden of Disease: 2004 Update. WHO; 2008
2 Lake, J., & Turner, M. S. (2017). Urgent Need for Improved Mental Health Care and a More Collaborative Model of Care. *The Permanente journal*, 21, 17–024. https://doi.org/10.7812/TPP/17-024

3 Depression: Fact sheet [Internet] Geneva, Switzerland: World Health Organization; updated 2017 Feb [cited 2017 Jun 15]. Available from: www.who.int/mediacentre/factsheets/fs369/en/

4 Bhui, K., Dinos, S., Galant-Miecznikowska, M., de Jongh, B., & Stansfeld, S. (2016). Perceptions of work stress causes and effective interventions in employees working in public, private and non-governmental organisations: a qualitative study. *BJPsych bulletin*, 40(6), 318–325. https://doi.org/10.1192/pb.bp.115.050823

5 Sharpless, B. A., & Barber, J. P. (2011). A Clinician's Guide to PTSD Treatments for Returning Veterans. *Professional psychology, research and practice*, 42(1), 8–15. https://doi.org/10.1037/a00223510004969172.INDD 19 10/13/2020 12:49:10 PM20 How to promote wellbeing

6 Henderson, C., Evans-Lacko, S., & Thornicroft, G. (2013). Mental illness stigma, help seeking, and public health programs. *American journal of public health*, 103(5), 777–780. https://doi.org/10.2105/AJPH.2012.301056

7 Mental health action plan 2013–2020 [Internet] Geneva, Switzerland: World Health Organization; 2013. [cited 2017 Jun 16]. Available from: http://apps.who.int/iris/bitstream/10665/89966/1/9789241506021_eng.pdf.

8 Spiers, J., Buszewicz, M., Chew-Graham, C., Gerada, C., Kessler, D., Leggett, N., Manning, C., Taylor, A., Thornton, G., & Riley, R. (2016). Who cares for the clinicians? The mental health crisis in the GP workforce. *The British journal of general practice : the journal of the Royal College of General Practitioners*, 66(648), 344–345. https://doi.org/10.3399/bjgp16X685765

9 Borrell-Carrió, F., Suchman, A. L., & Epstein, R. M. (2004). The biopsychosocial model 25 years later: principles, practice, and scientific inquiry. *Annals of family medicine*, 2(6), 576-82.

10 Tripathi, A., Das, A., & Kar, S. K. (2019). Biopsychosocial Model in Contemporary Psychiatry: Current Validity and Future Prospects. *Indian journal of psychological medicine*, 41(6), 582–585. https://doi.org/10.4103/IJPSYM.IJPSYM_314_19

11 Schneiderman, N., Ironson, G., & Siegel, S. D. (2005). Stress and health: psychological, behavioral, and biological determinants. *Annual review of clinical psychology*, 1, 607–628. doi:10.1146/annurev.clinpsy.1.102803.144141

12 Yaribeygi, H., Panahi, Y., Sahraei, H., Johnston, T. P., & Sahebkar, A. (2017). The impact of stress on body function: A review. *EXCLI journal*, 16, 1057–1072. https://doi.org/10.17179/excli2017-480

13 Godoy, L. D., Rossignoli, M. T., Delfino-Pereira, P., Garcia-Cairasco, N., & de Lima Umeoka, E. H. (2018). A Comprehensive Overview on Stress Neurobiology: Basic Concepts and Clinical Implications. *Frontiers in behavioral neuroscience*, 12, 127. https://doi.org/10.3389/fnbeh.2018.00127

14 Arnsten, A. F. (2009). Stress signalling pathways that impair prefrontal cortex structure and function. *Nature reviews. Neuroscience*, 10(6), 410–422. https://doi.org/10.1038/nrn2648

15 https://www.clinicalservicesjournal.com/story/25462/healthcare-hasthird-most-stressed-workers-in-uk

16 Shansky, R.M., & Lipps, J. (2013) Stress-induced cognitive dysfunction: hormone-neurotransmitter interactions in the prefrontal cortex *Front. Hum. Neurosci.*, https://doi.org/10.3389/fnhum.2013.00123

17 Arnau-Soler, A., Adams, M. J., Clarke, T. K., MacIntyre, D. J., Milburn, K., Navrady, L., C., McIntosh, A., & Thomson, P. A. (2019). Generation Scotland, Major Depressive Disorder Working Group of the Psychiatric Genomics Consortium, Hayward, A validation of the diathesis-stress model for depression in Generation Scotland. *Translational psychiatry*, 9(1), 25. https://doi.org/10.1038/s41398-018-0356-7

18 Mazure, C.M. (1998) Life stressors as risk factors in depression. *Clin. Psychol.* 5:291–313.

19 Lai, J., Ma, S. et al. (2019). Factors associated with mental health outcomes among health care workers exposed to Coronavirus Disease. *JAMA Netw Open* 2020;3:e203976

20 Rössler, W. (2016). The stigma of mental disorders: A millennia-long history of social exclusion and prejudices. *EMBO reports*, 17(9), 1250–1253. https://doi.org/10.15252/embr.201643041

21 Knaak, S., Mantler, E., & Szeto, A. (2017). Mental illness-related stigma in healthcare: Barriers to access and care and evidence-based solutions. *Healthcare management forum*, 30(2), 111–116. https://doi.org/10.1177/0840470416679413

22 https://jamanetwork.com/channels/health-forum/fullarticle/2764228

23 Greenberg, N., Docherty, M. et al. (2020) Managing mental health challenges faced by healthcare workers during covid-19 pandemic. *BMJ* 368:m12110004969172. INDD 21 10/13/2020 12:49:10 PM

Chapter 2

1 Spiers, J., Buszewicz, M., Chew-Graham, C., Gerada, C., Kessler, D., Leggett, N., Manning, C., Taylor, A., Thornton, G., & Riley, R. (2016). Who cares for the clinicians? The mental health crisis in the GP workforce. *The British journal of general practice : the journal of the Royal College of General Practitioners*, 66(648), 344–345. doi:10.3399/bjgp16X685765

2 The Bible, Luke 4:23 (King James version).

3 Center, C., Davis, M., Detre, T., Ford, D.E., Hansbrough, W., Hendin, H., Laszlo, J., Litts, D.A., Mann, J., Mansky, P.A., Michels, R., Miles, S.H., Proujansky, R., Reynolds, C.F. 3rd, & Silverman, M.M. (2003) Confronting depression and suicide in physicians: a consensus statement. *JAMA*. Jun 18; 289(23):3161–6.

4 Sheikhmoonesi, F., & Zarghami, M. (2014). Prevention of physicians' suicide. *Iranian journal of psychiatry and behavioral sciences*, 8(2), 1–3.

5 Hem, E., Haldorsen, T., Aasland, O.G., Tyssen, R., Vaglum, P., & Ekeberg, O. (2005) Suicide rates according to education with a particular focus on physicians in Norway 1960-2000. *Psychol Med*. Jun;35(6):873-80.

6 Daneault, S. (2008). The wounded healer: can this idea be of use to family physicians?. *Canadian family physician Medecin de famille canadien*, 54(9), 1218–1225.

7 Jung, C.(1951) *Fundamental questions of psychotherapy*. Princeton, NJ: Princeton University Press

8 Frankl, V. (1959) *Man's search for meaning*. New York, NY: Simon and Schuster

9   Widera, E., Chang, A., & Chen, H. L. (2010). Presenteeism: a public health hazard. *Journal of general internal medicine*, 25(11), 1244–1247. doi:10.1007/s11606-010-1422-x

10 Nagata, T., Mori, K., Ohtani, M., Nagata, M., Kajiki, S., Fujino, Y., Matsuda, S., & Loeppke, R. (2018) Total Health-Related Costs Due to Absenteeism, Presenteeism, and Medical and Pharmaceutical Expenses in Japanese Employers. *J Occup Environ Med.* May;60(5):e273-e280. doi: 10.1097/JOM.0000000000001291.

11 Turnberg, W., Daniell, W., & Duchin (2010) Influenza vaccination and sick leave practices and perceptions reported by health care workers in ambulatory care settings. *J Am J Infect Control.* Aug; 38(6):486–8.

12 Böckerman, P., & Laukkanen, E. (2010) What makes you work while you are sick? Evidence from a survey of workzers. *Eur J Public Health.* Feb; 20(1):43–6.

13 Vivancos, R., Sundkvist, T., Barker, D., Burton, J., & Nair, P. (2010) Effect of exclusion policy on the control of outbreaks of suspected viral gastroenteritis: Analysis of outbreak investigations in care homes. *Am J Infect Control.* Mar; 38(2):139–43.

14 Sarafis, P., Rousaki, E., Tsounis, A., Malliarou, M., Lahana, L., Bamidis, P., Niakas, D., & Papastavrou, E. (2016). The impact of occupational stress on nurses' caring behaviors and their health related quality of life. *BMC nursing,* 15, 56. https://doi.org/10.1186/s12912-016-0178-y

15 Norton, P., Costa, V., Teixeira J., Azevedo, A., Roma-Torres, A., Amaro, J., & Cunha, L. (2017) Prevalence and Determinants of Bullying Among Health Care Workers in Portugal. *Workplace Health Saf.* May;65(5):188-196. doi:10.1177/2165079916666545. Epub 2017 Jan 6.

16 Carter, M., Thompson, N., Crampton, P., Morrow, G., Burford, B., Gray, C., & Illing, J. (2013). Workplace bullying in the UK NHS: a questionnaire and interview study on prevalence, impact and barriers to reporting. *BMJ Open,* 3(6), e002628. https://doi.org/10.1136/bmjopen-2013-002628

17 Gandi, J. C., Wai, P. S., Karick, H., & Dagona, Z. K. (2011). The role of stress and level of burnout in job performance among nurses. *Mental health in family medicine,* 8(3), 181–194.

18 https://www.who.int/mental_health/evidence/burn-out/en/

19 https://icd.who.int/browse11/l-m/en#/http://id.who.int/icd/entity/129180281

20 https://www.wma.net/news-post/world-medical-association-welcomesdecision-on-burnout/0004969173.INDD 39 10/13/2020 12:52:42 PM

21 Freudenberger, H. (1974) Staff burnout. *J. Soc. Issues.*30:159–165. doi: 10.1111/j.1540-4560.1974.tb00706.x.

22 Maslach C., & Jackson S. (1986) Maslach Burnout Inventory manual. 2nd ed. Consulting Psychologist Press; Palo Alto, CA, USA

23 https://archive.bma.org.uk/news/media-centre/press-releases/2019/may/serious-mental-health-crisis-among-doctors-and-medical-students-revealed-inbma-report

24 Kumar, S. (2016). Burnout and Doctors: Prevalence, Prevention and Intervention. *Healthcare (Basel, Switzerland),* 4(3), 37. doi:10.3390/healthcare4030037

25 Shanafelt, T.D., Boone, S., Tan, L., Dyrbye, L.N., Sotile, W., Satele, D., West, C.P., Sloan, J., Oreskovich, M.R. (2012) Burnout and satisfaction with work-life balance among US physicians relative to the general US population. *Arch Intern Med.* Oct 8; 172(18):1377–85.

26 Thommasen, H.V., Lavanchy, M., Connelly, I., Berkowitz, J., & Grzybowski, S. (2001) Mental health, job satisfaction, and intention to relocate. Opinions of physicians in rural British Columbia. *Can Fam Physician*. Apr;47:737-44.

27 Sharma, A., Sharp, D.M., Walker, L.G., Monson, J.R. (2008) Stress and burnout in colorectal and vascular surgical consultants working in the UK National Health Service. *Psychooncology*. Jun;17(6):570 6.

28 Shanafelt, T.D., Balch, C.M., Bechamps, G., Russell, T., Dyrbye, L., Satele, D., Collicott, P., Novotny, P.J., Sloan, J., & Freischlag, J.(2010) Burnout and medical errors among American surgeons. *Ann Surg*. Jun;251(6):995-1000. doi: 10.1097/SLA.0b013e3181bfdab3.

29 Chipchase, S.Y., Chapman, H.R. & Bretherton, R. (2017) A study to explore if dentists' anxiety affects their clinical decision-making *BDJ* volume222, pages277–290 (24 February 2017)

30 Galletta, M., Portoghese, I., D'Aloja, E., Mereu, A., Contu, P., Coppola, R.C., Finco, G., Campagna, M. (2016) Relationship between job burnout, psychosocial factors and health care-associated infections in critical care units. *Intensive Crit Care Nurs*. Jun;34:51-8. doi: 10.1016/j.iccn.2015.11.004. Epub 2016 Mar 5.

31 Cimiotti, J. P., Aiken, L. H., Sloane, D. M., & Wu, E. S. (2012). Nurse staffing, burnout, and health care-associated infection. *American journal of infection control*, 40(6), 486–490. doi:10.1016/j.ajic.2012.02.029

32 Denton, D.A., Newton, J.T., Bower, E. J. (2008) Occupational burnout and work engagement: a national survey of dentists in the United Kingdom. *Br Dent J* 205, E13E13

33 Baer, T.E., Feraco, A.M., Tuysuzoglu, Sagalowsky, S., Williams, D., Litman, H.J., & Vinci, R.J. (2017) Pediatric Resident Burnout and Attitudes Toward Patients. *Pediatrics* Mar;139(3). pii: e20162163. doi: 10.1542/peds.2016-2163.

34 Chambers, C.N.L., Frampton, C.M.A., Barclay, M., et al (2016) Burnout prevalence in New Zealand's public hospital senior medical workforce: a cross-sectional mixed methods study BMJ Open;6:e013947.

35 Imo, U.O. (2017). Burnout and psychiatric morbidity among doctors in the UK: a systematic literature review of prevalence and associated factors. *BJPsych bulletin*, 41(4), 197–204.

36 Lo, D., Wu, F., Chan, M., Chu, R., & Li, D. (2018). A systematic review of burnout among doctors in China: a cultural perspective. *Asia Pacific family medicine*, 17, 3.

37 Bawakid, K., Abdulrashid, O., Mandoura, N., Shah, H., Ibrahim, A., Akkad, N. M., & Mufti, F. (2017). Burnout of Physicians Working in Primary Health Care Centers under Ministry of Health Jeddah, Saudi Arabia. *Cureus*, 9(11), e1877.

38 Kansoun, Z., Boyer, L., Hodgkinson, M., Villes, V., Lançon, C., & Fond, G. (2019) Burnout in French physicians: A systematic review and meta-analysis. *J Affect Disord*;246:132-147.

39 Rodrigues, H., Cobucci, R., Oliveira, A., Cabral, J.V., Medeiros, L., Gurgel, K., et al. (2018) Burnout syndrome among medical residents: A systematic review and meta-analysis. *PLoS ONE* 13(11): e0206840.

40 Peckham, C. (2017) Medscape Lifestyle Report 2017: race and ethnicity, bias and burnout. Medscape Lifestyle Report

41 Rossouw, L., Seedat, S., Emsley, R.A., Suliman, S. & Hagemeister, D. (2013) The prevalence of burnout and depression in medical doctors working in the Cape Town Metropolitan Municipality community healthcare clinics and district hospitals of the Provincial Government of the Western Cape: a cross-sectional study, *South African Family Practice*, 55:6, 567-573

42 Parr, J. M., Pinto, N., Hanson, M., Meehan, A., & Moore, P. T. (2016). Medical Graduates, Tertiary Hospitals, and Burnout: A Longitudinal Cohort Study. *The Ochsner journal*, 16(1), 22–26.

43 Zuraida, A.S., Zainal, N.Z. (2015) Exploring burnout among Malaysian junior doctors using the abbreviated Maslach Burnout Inventory. *Malaysian J Psych.* 2015;24(1):1–10. http://mjpsychiatry.org/index.php/mjp/article/view/348

44 Meier, D.E., Back, A.L., & Morrison, R.S. (2001) The inner life of physicians and care of the seriously ill. Dec 19; *JAMA*. 286(23):3007–14.

45 Myers, M.F. (2008) Physician impairment: is it relevant to academic psychiatry? *Acad Psychiatry*. Jan-Feb; 32(1):39–43.

46 https://www.medicalprotection.org/uk/articles/urgent-action-needed-to-tackleburnout-endemic-in-healthcare

47 Hughes, D., Burke, D., Hickie, I., Wilson, A., & Tobin M. (2002) Advanced training in adult psychiatry. *Australas. Psychiatry*. 10:6–11. doi: 10.1046/j.1440-1665.2002.00384.x

48 Cocker, F., & Joss, N. (2016). Compassion Fatigue among Healthcare, Emergency and Community Service Workers: A Systematic Review. *International journal of environmental research and public health*, 13(6), 618. https://doi.org/10.3390/ijerph13060618

49 Stamm, B.H. (2010) The Concise Proqol Manual. 2nd ed. Proqol.org; Pocatello, ID, USA:

50 Zhang, Y. Y., Zhang, C., Han, X. R., Li, W., & Wang, Y. L. (2018). Determinants of compassion satisfaction, compassion fatigue and burn out in nursing: A correlative meta-analysis. *Medicine*, 97(26), e11086. https://doi.org/10.1097/MD.0000000000011086

51 Sanchez-Reilly, S., Morrison, L. J., Carey, E., Bernacki, R., O'Neill, L., Kapo, J., Periyakoil, V. S., & Thomas, J. (2013). Caring for oneself to care for others: physicians and their self-care. *The journal of supportive oncology*, 11(2), 75–81. https://doi.org/10.12788/j.suponc.0003

52 Middleton, J. (2015) Addressing secondary trauma and compassion fatigue in work with older veterans: An ethical imperative, *Aging Life Care J.* 5;5:1, 8

53 Valent, P. (2002) Diagnosis and treatment of helper stresses, traumas, and illnesses; Treating Compassion Fatigue. Brunner-Routledge; New York City, NY, USA: pp. 17–37.

54 Peters, M. & King, J. (2012). Perfectionism in doctors. *BMJ (Clinical research ed.)*. 344. e1674. 10.1136/bmj.e1674.

55 Flett, G. (2004) York researcher finds that perfectionism can lead to imperfect health. File York's Daily Bulletin, York University, Toronto, Canada, June

56 Henning, K., Ey, S., Shaw, D. (1998) Perfectionism, the imposter phenomenon and psychological adjustment in medical, dental, nursing and pharmacy students. *Med Educ*. Sep; 32(5):456–64.

57   Boivin, D.B., & Boudreau, P. (2014) Impacts of shift work on sleep and circadian rhythms. *Pathol Biol* (Paris). Oct;62(5):292-301. doi: 10.1016/j.patbio.2014.08.001. Epub 2014 Sep 20.

58   Ferri, P., Guadi, M., Marcheselli, L., Balduzzi, S., Magnani, D., & Di Lorenzo, R. (2016). The impact of shift work on the psychological and physical health of nurses in a general hospital: a comparison between rotating night shifts and day shifts. *Risk management and healthcare policy*, 9, 203–211. doi:10.2147/RMHP. S115326

59   McVicar, A. (2016). Scoping the common antecedents of job stress and job satisfaction for nurses (2000-2013) using the job demands-resources model of stress. *J Nurs Manag*. (2016) Mar;24(2):E112-36. doi: 10.1111/jonm.12326. Epub 2015 Jul 14.

Chapter 3

1   Huffman, J. C., Celano, C. M., Beach, S. R., Motiwala, S. R., & Januzzi, J. L. (2013). Depression and cardiac disease: epidemiology, mechanisms, and diagnosis. *Cardiovascular psychiatry and neurology*, 2013, 695925. doi:10.1155/2013/695925

2   Wulsin, L. R., & Singal, B. M. (2003). Do depressive symptoms increase the risk for the onset of coronary disease? A systematic quantitative review. *Psychosomatic medicine*, 65(2), 201–210. https://doi.org/10.1097/01.psy.0000058371.50240.e3

3   Teh, C. F., Zaslavsky, A. M., Reynolds, C. F., 3rd, & Cleary, P. D. (2009). Effect of depression treatment on chronic pain outcomes. *Psychosomatic medicine*, 72(1), 61–67. doi:10.1097/PSY.0b013e3181c2a7a8

4   von Leupoldt, A., Taube, K., Lehmann, K., Fritzsche, A., & Magnussen, H. (2011). The impact of anxiety and depression on outcomes of pulmonary rehabilitation in patients with COPD. *Chest*, 140(3), 730–736. https://doi.org/10.1378/chest.10-2917

5   https://patient.info/doctor/screening-for-depression-in-primary-care

6   https://patient.info/doctor/patient-health-questionnaire-phq-9

7   Vogel, D., Meyer, M., & Harendza, S. (2018). Verbal and non-verbal communication skills including empathy during history taking of undergraduate medical students. *BMC medical education*, 18(1), 157. https://doi.org/10.1186/s12909-018-1260-9

8   Grace, G. D., & Christensen, R. C. (2007). Recognizing psychologically masked illnesses: the need for collaborative relationships in mental health care. *Primary care companion to the Journal of clinical psychiatry*, 9(6), 433–436. https://doi.org/10.4088/pcc.v09n0605

9   Osborn, D. P. (2001). The poor physical health of people with mental illness. *The Western journal of medicine*, 175(5), 329–332. https://doi.org/10.1136/ewjm.175.5.329

10   Besedovsky, L., Lange, T., & Born, J. (2012). Sleep and immune function. *Pflugers Archiv : European journal of physiology*, 463(1), 121–137. https://doi.org/10.1007/s00424-011-1044-0

11   McLain, J. M., Alami, W. H., Glovak, Z. T., Cooley, C. R., Burke, S. J., Collier, J. J., Baghdoyan, H. A., Karlstad, M. D., & Lydic, R. (2018). Sleep fragmentation delays

wound healing in a mouse model of type 2 diabetes. *Sleep,* 41(11), *zsy156*. https://doi.org/10.1093/sleep/zsy156

12 Tosini, G., Ferguson, I., & Tsubota, K. (2016). Effects of blue light on the circadian system and eye physiology. *Molecular vision,* 22, 61–72.

13 Russell, L. (2001) The importance of patients' nutritional status in wound healing. *Br J Nurs.* Mar;10(6 Suppl):S42, S44-9.

Chapter 4

1 Panagioti, M., Panagopoulou, E., Bower, P., Lewith, G., Kontopantelis, E., Chew-Graham, C., Dawson, S., van Marwijk, H., Geraghty, K., & Esmail, A. (2017) Controlled Interventions to Reduce Burnout in Physicians: A Systematic Review and Meta-analysis. *JAMA Intern Med.* Feb 1;177(2):195-205. doi: 10.1001/jamainternmed.2016.7674.

2 Cook, R.I., Render, M., Woods, D.D. (2000) Gaps: learning how practitioners create safety. *BMJ* 320:791–4.

3 Jeffcott, S.A., Ibrahim, J.E. & Cameron, P.A. (2009) Resilience in healthcare and clinical handover. *Qual Saf Health Care* 18: 256–260 doi: 10.1136/qshc.2008.030163

4 Wears, R. L. (2006). Resilience Engineering: Concepts and Precepts. *Quality & Safety in Health Care,* 15(6), 447–448. doi:10.1136/qshc.2006.018390

5 Bomba, D.T., & Prakash R (2005) A description of handover processes in an Australian public hospital. *Aust Health Rev.* Feb;29(1):68–79.

6 Spiers, J., Buszewicz, M., Chew-Graham, C., Gerada, C., Kessler, D., Leggett, N., Manning, C., Taylor, A., Thornton, G., & Riley, R. (2016). Who cares for the clinicians? The mental health crisis in the GP workforce. *The British journal of general practice : the journal of the Royal College of General Practitioners,* 66(648), 344–345. https://doi.org/10.3399/bjgp16X685765

7 Knaak, S., Mantler, E., & Szeto, A. (2017). Mental illness-related stigma in healthcare: Barriers to access and care and evidence-based solutions. *Healthcare management forum,* 30(2), 111–116. https://doi.org/10.1177/0840470416679413

8 https://archive.bma.org.uk/collective-voice/policy-and-research/educationtraining-and-workforce/supporting-the-mental-health-of-doctors-in-theworkforce

9 https://www.bma.org.uk/collective-voice/policy-and-research/education-trainingand-workforce/supporting-the-mental-health-of-doctors-in-theworkforce

10 https://archive.bma.org.uk/news/media-centre/press-releases/2019/october/employers-must-address-mental-health-crisis-among-doctors-and-provideworkplace-support-says-bma

11 Vermeir, P., Vandijck, D., Degroote, S., Peleman, R., Verhaeghe, R., Mortier, E., Hallaert, G., Van Daele, S., Buylaert, W., & Vogelaers, D. (2015). Communication in healthcare: a narrative review of the literature and practical recommendations. *International journal of clinical practice,* 69(11), 1257–1267. https://doi.org/10.1111/ijcp.12686

12 https://www.gmc-uk.org/education/standards-guidance-and-curricula/guidance/reflective-practice/schwartz-rounds

13 https://www.pointofcarefoundation.org.uk/blog/enabling-and-supporting-staffto-care-well/ -

14 https://www.journalslibrary.nihr.ac.uk/programmes/hsdr/130749/#/

15 https://www.gmc-uk.org/education/standards-guidance-and-curricula/guidance/reflective-practice/balint-groups

16 Dollard, M.F., & McTernan, W. (2011) Psychosocial safety climate: a multilevel theory of work stress in the health and community service sector. *Epidemiol Psychiatr Sci.* Dec;20(4):287–93.

17 Iavicoli, S., Cesana, G., Dollard, M., Leka, S., & Sauter, S. L. (2015). Psychosocial Factors and Workers' Health and Safety. *BioMed research international,* 628749. doi:10.1155/2015/628749

18 Law, R., Dollard, M.F., Tuckey, M.R., & Dormann, C. (2011) Psychosocial safety climate as a lead indicator of workplace bullying and harassment, job resources, psychological health and employee engagement. *Accid Anal Prev.* Sep;43(5):1782–93. doi: 10.1016/j.aap.2011.04.010. Epub 2011 May 4.

19 Hall, G.B., Dollard, M.F., Winefield, A.H., Dormann, C., & Bakker, A.B. (2013) Psychosocial safety climate buffers effects of job demands on depression and positive organizational behaviors, *Anxiety Stress Coping,* 26(4):355–77. doi: 10.1080/10615806.2012.700477. Epub 2012 Jul 16.

20 Maslach, C., & Leiter, M. (1999) Six areas of work life: A model of the organisational context of burnout, *Journal of health and human services administration* 21(4): 471–489

Chapter 5

1 Center for Substance Abuse Treatment. Enhancing Motivation for Change in Substance Abuse Treatment. Rockville (MD): Substance Abuse and Mental Health Services Administration (US); 1999. (Treatment Improvement Protocol (TIP) Series, No. 35.) Chapter 1-- Conceptualizing Motivation And Change. Available from: https://www.ncbi.nlm.nih.gov/books/NBK64972/

2 Miller, W. R., & Rose, G. S. (2009). Toward a theory of motivational interviewing. *The American psychologist,* 64(6), 527–537. doi:10.1037/a0016830

3 Wu, G., Feder, A., Cohen, H., Kim, J. J., Calderon, S., Charney, D. S., & Mathé, A. A. (2013). Understanding resilience. *Frontiers in behavioral neuroscience,* 7, 10. doi:10.3389/fnbeh.2013.00010

4 Oshioa, A., Takub, K., Hiranoc, M., & Saeedd, G. (2018) Resilience and Big Five personality traits: A meta- analysis. *Personality and Individual Differences Volume* 127, Pages 54–60

5 Sull, A., Harland, N., & Moore, A. (2015). Resilience of health-care workers in the UK; a cross-sectional survey. *Journal of occupational medicine and toxicology* 10, 20. doi:10.1186/s12995-015-0061-x

6 Violanti, J. M., Fekedulegn, D., Hartley, T. A., Andrew, M. E., Charles, L., Tinney-Zara, C. A., & Burchfiel, C. M. (2014). Police Work Absence: An Analysis of Stress and Resiliency. *Journal of law enforcement leadership and ethics,* 1(1), 49–67.

7 Zhang, Y. Y., Zhang, C., Han, X. R., Li, W., & Wang, Y. L. (2018). Determinants of compassion satisfaction, compassion fatigue and burn out in nursing: A correlative

meta-analysis. *Medicine,* 97(26), e11086. https://doi.org/10.1097/MD.0000000000011086

8 Walker, H.K., Hall, W.D., & Hurst, J.W. (1990) Clinical Methods: The History, Physical, and Laboratory Examinations. 3rd edition.Boston: Butterworths

9 Nolte, A.G., Downing, C., Temane, A., & Hastings-Tolsma, M. (2017) Compassion fatigue in nurses: A metasynthesis. *J Clin Nurs.* Dec; 26(23-24):4364–4378.

10 Alkema, K., Linton, J.M., & Davies, R. (2008) A study of the relationship between self-care, compassion satisfaction, compassion fatigue, and burnout among hospice professionals. *J Soc Work End Life Palliat Care.* 4(2):101–19.

11 Sanchez-Reilly, S., Morrison, L. J., Carey, E., Bernacki, R., O'Neill, L., Kapo, J., Periyakoil, V. S., & Thomas, J. (2013). Caring for oneself to care for others: physicians and their self-care. *The journal of supportive oncology,* 11(2), 75–81. https://doi.org/10.12788/j.suponc.0003

12 Wallace, J.E., Lemaire, J.B., & Ghali, W.A. (2009) Physician wellness: a missing quality indicator. *Lancet.* Nov 14; 374(9702):1714–21.

13 Wiskow C., Albreht T., de Pietro C (2010) How to Create an Attractive and Supportive Working Environment for Health Professionals.WHO; *Copenhagen, Denmark*: 2010. pp. 1–37.

14 Amoafo, E., Hanbali, N., Patel, A., Singh, P. (2015). What are the significant factors associated with burnout in doctors? *Occup Med (Lond).* Mar; 65(2):117–21.

15 https://www.bma.org.uk/collective-voice/policy-and-research/education-trainingand-workforce/suppor ting-the-mental-health-of-doctors-in-theworkforce#principles

16 Dyrbye, L.N., Shanafelt, T.D., Balch, C.M., Satele, D., Sloan, J., & Freischlag (2011). Relationship between work-home conflicts and burnout among American surgeons: a comparison by sex. *J Arch Surg.* Feb; 146(2):211–7.

17 Bressi, C., Porcellana, M., Gambini, O., Madia, L., Muffatti, R., Peirone, A., Zanini, S., Erlicher, A., Scarone, S., & Altamura, A.C. (2009). Burnout among psychiatrists in Milan: a multicenter survey. *Psychiatr Serv.* Jul; 60(7):985–8.

18 https://news.doctors.net.uk/news/29760?utm_source=Bulletin&utm_medium=Email&utm_campaign=DNB

19 https://www.heti.nsw.gov.au/resources-and-links/covid-19/wellbeing/caring-for-your-team

20 Slavich, G. M., & Irwin, M. R. (2014). From stress to inflammation and major depressive disorder: a social signal transduction theory of depression. *Psychological bulletin,* 140(3), 774–815. doi:10.1037/a0035302

21 https://www.practitionerhealth.nhs.uk/about-practitioner-health

22 https://www.practitionerhealth.nhs.uk/treatment

23 Ahmed, J., Mehmood, S., Rehman, S., Ilyas, C., & Khan, L.U. (2012). Impact of a structured template and staff training on compliance and quality of clinical handover. *Int J Surg.* 10(9):571–4. doi: 10.1016/j.ijsu.2012.09.001. Epub 2012 Sep 13.

24 Sharma, H. (2015). Meditation: Process and effects. *Ayu,* 36(3), 233–237. doi:10.4103/0974-8520.182756

25 Goyal, M., Singh, S., Sibinga, E.M.S., et al. (2014). Meditation Programs for Psychological Stress and Well-Being Agency for Healthcare Research and Quality

(US); 2014 Jan. (Comparative Effectiveness Reviews, No. 124.) Available from: https://www.ncbi.nlm.nih.gov/books/NBK180102/

26 Elder, C., Nidich, S., Moriarty, F., & Nidich, R. (2014). Effect of Transcendental Meditation on employee stress, depression, and burnout: A randomized controlled study. *Perm J.* 2014;18:19–23.

27 Chen, K.W., Berger, C.C., Manheimer, E., Forde, D., Magidson, J., Dachman, L., & Lejuez, C.W. (2012) . Meditative therapies for reducing anxiety: a systematic review and metaanalysis of randomized controlled trials. *Depress Anxiety.* Jul; 29(7):545–62

28 Kasala, E.R., Bodduluru, L.N., Maneti, Y., & Thipparaboina, R. (2014). Effect of meditation on neurophysiological changes in stress mediated depression. *Complement Ther Clin Pract.* 20:74–80.

29 Orme-Johnson, D.W., Schneider, R.H., Son, Y.D., Nidich, S., & Cho, Z.H. (2006) Neuroimaging of meditation's effect on brain reactivity to pain. *Neuroreport.* Aug 21; 17(12):1359–63.

30 Khalsa, D.S. (2015) Stress, Meditation, and Alzheimer's Disease Prevention: Where The Evidence Stands. *J Alzheimers Dis.* 48(1):1–12.

31 Chan, D., & Woollacott, M. (2007) Effects of level of meditation experience on attentional focus: is the efficiency of executive or orientation networks improved? *J Altern Complement Med.* Jul-Aug; 13(6):651–7.

32 Rainforth, M.V., Schneider, R.H., Nidich, S.I., Gaylord-King, C., Salerno, J.W., & Anderson, J.W. (2007) Stress reduction programs in patients with elevated blood pressure: a systematic review and meta-analysis. *Curr Hypertens Rep.* Dec; 9(6):520–8.

33 Infante, J.R., Torres-Avisbal, M., Pinel, P., Vallejo, J.A., Peran, F., Gonzalez, F., Contreras, P., Pacheco, C., Roldan, A., & Latre, J.M. (2001) Catecholamine levels in practitioners of the transcendental meditation technique. *Physiol Behav.* Jan; 72(1-2):141–6.

34 Telles, S., Raghavendra, B.R., Naveen, K.V., Manjunath, N.K., Kumar, S., & Subramanya, P. (2013) Changes in autonomic variables following two meditative states described in yoga texts. *J Altern Complement Med.* Jan; 19(1):35–42.

35 Jevning, R., Anand, R., Biedebach, M., & Fernando, G. (1996). Effects on regional cerebral blood flow of Transcendental Meditation. *Physiol Behav.* 59:399–402.

36 Wallace, R.K., Dillbeck, M., Jacobe, E., & Harrington, B. (1982) The effects of the transcendental meditation and TM-Sidhi program on the aging process. *Int J Neurosci. Feb*; 16(1):53–8.

37 Kabat-Zinn, J. (1994) *Wherever you go, there you are: mindfulness meditation in everyday life.* New York (NY): Hyperion

38 Hoge, E. A., Bui, E., Marques, L., Metcalf, C. A., Morris, L. K., Robinaugh, D. J., & Simon, N. M. (2013). Randomized controlled trial of mindfulness meditation for generalized anxiety disorder: effects on anxiety and stress reactivity. *The Journal of clinical psychiatry,* 74(8), 786–792. doi:10.4088/JCP.12m08083

39 Chiesa, A., & Serretti, A. (2009) *J* Mindfulness-based stress reduction for stress management in healthy people: a review and meta-analysis. *Altern Complement Med.* May; 15(5):593–600.

40 Goldin, P. R., & Gross, J. J. (2010). Effects of mindfulness-based stress reduction (MBSR) on emotion regulation in social anxiety disorder. *Emotion* 10(1), 83–91. doi:10.1037/a0018441

41 Segal, Z.V., Williams, J.M.G., & Teasdale, J.D. (2002) *Mindfulness-based cognitive therapy for depression — a new approach to preventing relapse.* New York (NY): Guilford Press

42 Young, S. N. (2011). Biologic effects of mindfulness meditation: growing insights into neurobiologic aspects of the prevention of depression. *Journal of psychiatry & neuroscience: JPN,* 36(2), 75–77. doi:10.1503/jpn.110010

43 Gooley, J. J., Chamberlain, K., Smith, K. A., Khalsa, S. B., Rajaratnam, S. M., Van Reen, E., & Lockley, S. W. (2010). Exposure to room light before bedtime suppresses melatonin onset and shortens melatonin duration in humans. *The Journal of clinical endocrinology and metabolism,* 96(3), E463–E472. doi:10.1210/jc.2010-2098

44 Ribeiro, J.A., & Sebastião, A.M. (2010) Caffeine and adenosine. *J Alzheimers Dis.* 20 Suppl 1:S3-15. doi: 10.3233/JAD-2010-1379.

45 Bjorness, T. E., & Greene, R. W. (2009). Adenosine and sleep. *Current neuropharmacology,* 7(3), 238–245. doi:10.2174/157015909789152182

46 Caffeine for the Sustainment of Mental Task Performance: Formulations for Military Operations (2001) Institute of Medicine (US) Committee on Military Nutrition Research. Washington (DC): National Academies Press (US)

47 Lovato, N., & Lack, L. (2010) The effects of napping on cognitive functioning. *Prog Brain Res.* 185:155–66. doi: 10.1016/B978-0-444-53702-7.00009-9.

48 Owens, J.F., Buysse, D.J., Hall, M., Kamarck, T.W., Lee, L., Strollo, P.J., Reis, S.E., & Matthews, K.A. (2010) Napping, Nighttime Sleep, and Cardiovascular Risk Factors in Mid-Life Adults. *J Clin Sleep Med.* Aug 15; 6(4): 330–335.

49 Okamoto-Mizuno, K., & Mizuno, K. (2012). Effects of thermal environment on sleep and circadian rhythm. *Journal of physiological anthropology,* 31(1), 14. doi:10.1186/1880-6805-31-14

50 Nutt, D., Wilson, S., & Paterson, L. (2008). Sleep disorders as core symptoms of depression. *Dialogues in clinical neuroscience,* 10(3), 329–336.

51 Scholey, A.B., Harper, S.,& Kennedy, D.O. (2001). Cognitive demand and blood glucose. *Physiol Behav.* Jul;73(4):585–92.

52 Manning, C.A., Parsons, M.W., Cotter, E.M., & Gold, P.E. (1997). Glucose effects on declarative and non-declarative memory in healthy elderly and young adults. *Psychobiology.* 25:103–8

53 Graveling, A. J., Deary, I. J., & Frier, B. M. (2013). Acute hypoglycemia impairs executive cognitive function in adults with and without type 1 diabetes. *Diabetes care,* 36(10), 3240–3246. doi:10.2337/dc13-0194

54 Philippou, E., & Constantinou, M. (2014). The influence of glycemic index on cognitive functioning: a systematic review of the evidence. *Advances in nutrition* 5(2), 119–130. doi:10.3945/an.113.004960

55 Eleazu, C. O. (2016). The concept of low glycemic index and glycemic load foods as panacea for type 2 diabetes mellitus; prospects, challenges and solutions. *African health sciences,* 16(2), 468–479. doi:10.4314/ahs.v16i2.15

56 Deepa, G., Singh, V., & Naidu, K.A. (2010). A comparative study on starch digesti-bility, glycemic index and resistant starch of pigmented ('Njavara' and 'Jyothi') and a non-pigmented ('IR 64') rice varieties. *J Food Sci Technol*. Dec; 47(6):644–9.

57 Brand-Miller, J.C. (2003) Glycemic load and chronic disease. *Nutr Rev*. May; 61(5 Pt 2):S49–55.

58 McGregor, S. J., Nicholas, C. W., Lakomy, H.K. et al (1999) The influence of inter-mittent high intensity shuttle running and fluid ingestion on the performances of a soccer skill. *J Sports Sci* 17895–903.

59 Suhr, J.A., Hall, J., Patterson, S.M., Niinistö, R.T. (2004). The relation of hydration status to cognitive performance in healthy older adults. *Int J Psychophysiol*. Jul; 53(2):121–5.

60 Maughan, R.J., Griffin, J. (2003) Caffeine ingestion and fluid balance: a review. *J Hum Nutr Diet*. Dec;16(6):411–20.

61 Nehlig, A. (2010) Is caffeine a cognitive enhancer? *J Alzheimers Dis*. 20 Suppl 1:S85–94. doi: 10.3233/JAD-2010-091315.

62 Melrose, S. (2011). Perfectionism and depression: vulnerabilities nurses need to understand. *Nursing research and practice*, 858497. doi:10.1155/2011/858497

63 Sturman, E.D., Flett, G.L., Hewitt, P.L., & Rudolph, S.G. (2009) Dimensions of perfectionism and self-worth contingencies in depression. *Journal of Rational-Emotive and Cognitive-Behavior Therapy*. 27(4):213–231.

64 Olson, M.L., & Kwon, P. (2008) Brooding perfectionism: refining the roles of rumination and perfectionism in the etiology of depression. *Cognitive Therapy and Research*. 32(6):788–802.

65 https://improvement.nhs.uk/documents/2265/Revised_Never_Events_policy_and_framework_FINAL.pdf

66 Never Events. Never Events list 2018. https://improvement.nhs.uk/documents/2899/never_events_list_2018_final_v6.pdf, NHS Improvements 2018. Licenced under CC-BY-Open Government License v3.0

67 Esonis, S. (2007) It's Your Little Red Wagon: 6 Core Strengths for Navigating Your Path to the Good Life. San Diego, Calif, USA: Positive Path Publishing

68 Lee, Y. H., Heeter, C., Magerko, B., & Medler, B. (2012). Gaming mindsets: implicit theories in serious game learning. *Cyberpsychology, behavior and social network-ing*, 15(4), 190–194. doi:10.1089/cyber.2011.0328

69 Ng, B. (2018). The Neuroscience of Growth Mindset and Intrinsic Motivation. *Brain sciences*, 8(2), 20. https://doi.org/10.3390/brainsci8020020

70 https://www.webmd.com/depression/guide/cognitive-behavioral-therapyfor-depression#1/

71 https://www.psychologytools.com/resource/living-with-worry-and-anxietyamidst-global-uncertainty

72 Neumann, T.A. (2010). Delegation-better safe than sorry. *AAOHN J*. Aug;58(8): 321–2.

73 Barrow, J.M., Sharma, S. (2020). Nursing Five Rights of Delegation Treasure Island (FL): StatPearls Publishing; Jan.

74 Blair, S.N., Kampert, J.B., Kohl, H.W. 3rd, Barlow, C.E., Macera, C.A., Paffenbarger, R.S. Jr., & Gibbons, L.W. (1996) Influences of cardiorespiratory fitness and other

precursors on cardiovascular disease and all-cause mortality in men and women. *JAMA*. Jul 17;276(3):205–10.

75 Zhao, M., Veeranki, S.P., Li, S., et al (2019) Beneficial associations of low and large doses of leisure time physical activity with all-cause, cardiovascular disease and cancer mortality: a national cohort study of 88,140 US adults *Br J Sports Med* Published Online First: 19 March 2019. doi: 10.1136/bjsports-2018-099254

76 Puterman, E., Lin, J., Blackburn, E., O'Donovan, A., Adler, N., & Epel, E. (2010) The Power of Exercise: Buffering the Effect of Chronic Stress on Telomere Length. *PLoS ONE* 5(5): e10837. https://doi.org/10.1371/journal.pone.0010837

77 Stults-Kolehmainen, M. A., & Sinha, R. (2014). The effects of stress on physical activity and exercise. *Sports medicine* (Auckland, N.Z.), 44(1), 81–121. doi:10.1007/s40279-013-0090-5

78 Seppälä, E. M., Nitschke, J. B., Tudorascu, D. L., Hayes, A., Goldstein, M. R., Nguyen, D. T. & Davidson, R. J. (2014). Breathing-based meditation decreases posttraumatic stress disorder symptoms in U.S. military veterans: a randomized controlled longitudinal study. *Journal of traumatic stress*, 27(4), 397–405. doi:10.1002/jts.21936

79 Prasad, L., Varrey, A., & Sisti, G. (2016). Medical Students' Stress Levels and Sense of Well Being after Six Weeks of Yoga and Meditation. *Evidence-based complementary and alternative medicine: eCAM*, 2016, 9251849. https://doi.org/10.1155/2016/9251849

80 Sansone, R. A., & Sansone, L. A. (2010). Gratitude and well being: the benefits of appreciation. *Psychiatry (Edgmont (Pa.: Township))*, 7(11), 18–22.

81 Emmons, R.A., & McCullough, M.E. (2003). Counting blessings versus burdens: an experimental investigation of gratitude and subjective well-being in daily life. *J Pers Soc Psychol*. Feb;84(2):377–89.

82 Froh, J.J., Sefick, W.J., & Emmons, R.A. (2008). Counting blessings in early adolescents: an experimental study of gratitude and subjective well-being. *J Sch Psychol*. Apr; 46(2):213–33.

83 Wood, A.M., Joseph, S., Lloyd, J., & Atkins, S. (2009) Gratitude influences sleep through the mechanism of pre-sleep cognitions. *J Psychosom Res*. Jan; 66(1):43–8

Chapter 6

1 Dyrbye, L.N., Sciolla, A.F., Dekhtyar, M., Rajasekaran, S., Allgood, J.A., Rea, M., Knight, A.P., Haywood, A., Smith, S., & Stephens, M.B. (2019) Medical School Strategies to Address Student Well-Being: A National Survey *Acad Med*. Jun;94(6):861-868. doi: 10.1097/ACM.0000000000002611..

2 Watling, C. (2015). Tackling medical student stress: beyond individual resilience. *Perspectives on medical education*, 4(3), 105–106. https://doi.org/10.1007/s40037-015-0190-z

3 Bloodgood, R.A., Short, J.G., Jackson, J.M., Martindale, J.R. (2009) A change to pass/fail grading in the first two years at one medical school results in improved psychological well-being. *Acad Med*. May; 84(5):655-62.

4 Park, S. G., & Park, K. H. (2018). Correlation between nonverbal communication and objective structured clinical examination score in medical students. *Korean journal of medical education*, 30(3), 199–208. https://doi.org/10.3946/kjme.2018.94

5 Burgoon, J.K., Guerrero, L.K., & Floyd, K. (2010) *Nonverbal communication*. Boston, USA: Pearson

6 Hall, J.A., Harrigan, J.A., & Rosenthal, R., (1995) Nonverbal behavior in clinician–patient interaction. *Appl Prev Psychol*. 4(1):21–37.

Chapter 7

1 Taber, J. M., Leyva, B., & Persoskie, A. (2014). Why do people avoid medical care? A qualitative study using national data. *Journal of general internal medicine*, 30(3), 290–297. doi:10.1007/s11606-014-3089-1

2 Greenberg, N., Docherty, M. et al (2020). Managing mental health challenges faced by healthcare workers during covid-19 pandemic. *BMJ* 368:m1211

3 https://www.hse.ie/eng/services/publications/mentalhealth/riskmanagement inmentalhealth.pdf

4 DesRoches, C.M., Rao, S.R., Fromson, J.A., Birnbaum, R.J., Iezzoni, L., Vogeli, C., & Campbell, E.G. (2010) Physicians' perceptions, preparedness for reporting, and experiences related to impaired and incompetent colleagues *JAMA*. 2010 Jul 14;304(2):187-93. doi: 10.1001/jama.2010.921..

5 White, C. (2004). Doctors mistrust systems for reporting medical mistakes. *BMJ: British Medical Journal*, 329(7456), 12.

6 https://www.england.nhs.uk/ourwork/whistleblowing/raising-a-concern/

7 Freestone, L., Bolsin, S.N., Colson, M., Patrick, A., & Creati, B. (2006) Voluntary incident reporting by anaesthetic trainees in an Australian hospital. *Int J Qual Health Care*. Dec;18(6):452-7. Epub 2006 Oct 19

8 Campbell, B., & Garner, S. (2008). NICE/NPSA patient safety pilot. *Annals of the Royal College of Surgeons of England*, 90(5), 439–440.doi:10.1308/003588408X301 280b

9 https://www.gov.uk/government/organisations/national-patient-safety-agency

10 Jane, C. (2009) Name and shame *BMJ* 339 :b2693

11 https://www.england.nhs.uk/ourwork/whistleblowing/raising-a-concern/

12 https://www.bma.org.uk/media/2217/bma-wellbeing-covid-19-poster.pdf

Index

How to Promote Wellbeing: Practical Steps for Healthcare Practitioners' Mental Health,
First Edition. Dr Rachel K Thomas.
© 2021 Dr Rachel K. Thomas. Published 2021 by John Wiley & Sons Ltd.